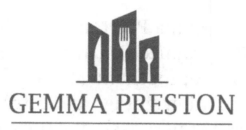

GEMMA PRESTON

COPYCAT RECIPES

MAKING THE MOST POPULAR SPAIN RECIPES AT HOME (FAMOUS RESTAURANT COPYCAT COOKBOOK)

GEMMA PRESTON

Copyright © Gemma Preston

Editing by Gemma Preston

Weekly Copycat Menu

Monday

....
....
....
....
....

Tuesday

....
....
....
....
....

Wednesday

....
....
....
....
....

Thursday

....
....
....
....
....

Friday

....
....
....
....
....

Saturday

....
....
....
....
....

Sunday

....
....
....
....
....

Snacks

....
....
....
....
....

Budget

....
....
....
....
....

Table of Content

Introduction

25 Spanish recipes to make at home.

If you are looking for ideas for a Hispanic dinner, here are 25 of the best recipes, churros and traditional Spanish tapas recipes.

Even Spanish cuisine, in recent years is highly sought after, one of the main reasons why I decided to write a book of Hispanic recipes is due to the fact that it is a purely Mediterranean cuisine and that goes hand in hand with different types of diets.

Spanish cuisine is very rich in culture and history, like the Italian one there are several regions that bring their own typical dish to the table. Cooking methods in Spain are simple: they reveal the delicious aromas and flavors of fresh ingredients.

Inside the cookbook you can indulge yourself with recipes ranging from meat to fish, from salads to desserts.

Impress your family or friends with the help of the cookbook, presenting your Spanish dishes, you will get a sense of gratification after having them savored by your loved ones.

After sharing some of the most popular Spanish dishes with you last week, I was inspired to show you how to prepare them. But since I'm not a food expert, I enlisted the help of real experts: food bloggers who surely know what they're talking about.

Here are 25 easy and authentic Spanish recipes you can make at home!

It comes close to keto cooking, in fact, in addition to the Spanish recipes, I wanted to include another 50 tasty keto recipes, consequently there are many dishes that you can use for a good ketogenic basic diet.

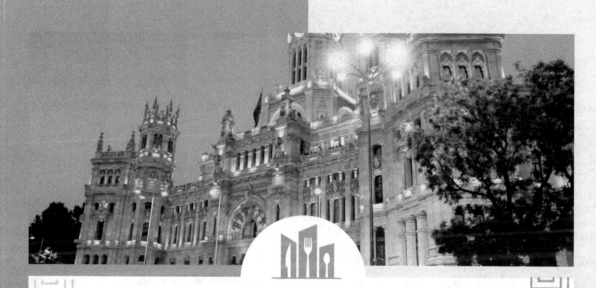

Copycat Recipes

MAKING THE MOST POPULAR SPANISH RECIPES AT HOME

FAMOUS RESTAURANT COPYCAT COOKBOOK

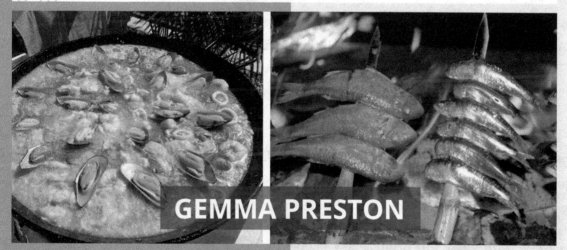

GEMMA PRESTON

Chapter 1. About (KETO) Cuisine

The Keto nutritional strategy is to consume high fat, moderate amounts of protein, and minimal carbs. It will help your body enter into the ketosis state, thereby resulting in the ketone bodies' production. Your body will soon turn into a fat-burning machine, helping you achieve your goal weight.

Remember, fat is an essential macronutrient that plays a significant role in the ketogenic diet, and it is not the fact that it makes you fat!

Cut carbs. The first and most vital step to take towards the Keto diet is cutting out carbs. I know it may sound straightforward, even trivial, but it's as tougher as it seems for most of us. The majority of us may have bread, pasta, potatoes, rice, or something similar at least once a day, but in a Keto diet, that has to be avoided. As someone who loves pasta, this was incredibly hard for me, but I managed, which paid off. We need to stay below 50 grams of carbs per day, ideally, down to 20 grams per day.

Limit protein. Now that we've cut out carbs, we need to replace them with the fatty foods that will power us when we reach ketosis. Many people make the mistake of replacing their carbs with protein, which is an issue because excess protein can be converted into glucose. If we have extra protein in our diet, we may find it harder to reach ketosis.

Avoid sugar. This diet may be a high-fat diet, but it doesn't mean sugary foods are good for us. Glucose, fructose, and sucrose are all incredibly common in candy, soft drinks, and junk food that you come across. These sugars are the exact things that we are trying to remove by cutting our diet's carbs. Besides natural sugars, we should also avoid sweeteners like xylitol, maltitol, aspartame, and saccharin. These sweeteners have similar net carbs to table sugar and should be avoided all the same.

Keep your vegetables above ground! Vegetables are an essential part of Keto, but we need to include only above-ground vegetables. Root vegetables are high in starch and sugars, while the vast majority of green vegetables are light on carbs. Some of the best vegetables for Keto diet include lettuce, spinach, asparagus, avocado, cauliflower, cucumber, and tomato.

Be careful with what you drink. Many people overlook their drinks while making diet, but we won't make that same mistake. In Keto diet, the drinks you have during the day can make or break your path to ketosis. Luckily, we have plenty of healthy options when it comes to refreshments.

We've all been taught since we were children that we should always drink plenty of water, and there isn't any reason for don't do that. Put slices of lemon or lime into your glass, and there you have a delicious drink with zero carbs. Tea and coffee are fantastic too, but avoid using any of the sugars or sweeteners mentioned above, and be careful using too much milk. Diet soft drinks can be fine as well, be careful to read the ingredients; many diet drinks may have sweeteners, which are still carb-heavy. Lastly, alcohol is very light on carbs; wine and pure spirits are all fine to drink in a Keto diet.

Increase healthy fats! As we've already read, the Keto diet is high-fat. As we've been taught to avoid fat for so many years, it is often hard to wrap our heads around needing more than 60% fat in our daily diet. Luckily, there are easy and healthy ways of increasing your fat intake. One tasty and easy to find a source of healthy fats is fish. Salmon, mackerel, herring, and sardines are great examples of fatty fish, all of which are easy to start and make for tasty meals. Another fantastic source of fats is oil. Coconut, avocado, and olive oil are healthy oil choices, which we can use for cooking meals and garnishing vegetables. Lastly, animal products are also a great way of filling out your healthy fats quota for the day. Eggs, cheese, butter, and cream can make perfect snacks throughout the day, especially when partnered with low carb nuts such as pecans, macadamias, and Brazil nuts.

Use a calorie counter. Even if you're following a detailed meal plan, keep a calorie counter with you. We must hold ourselves to the requirements of our Keto diet. Having an app or notepad that allows us to track our meals will help us learn more about our diet and reach our goals better.

New diets can be challenging initially, but the beauty about the Keto diet is that every change you need, makes it easily achievable. It's a series of small, manageable steps that lead to an incredible result. Take your time to work these changes into your daily life, and don't rush. Keto done at your own pace is the best kind of Keto.

2. Recipes from Spain

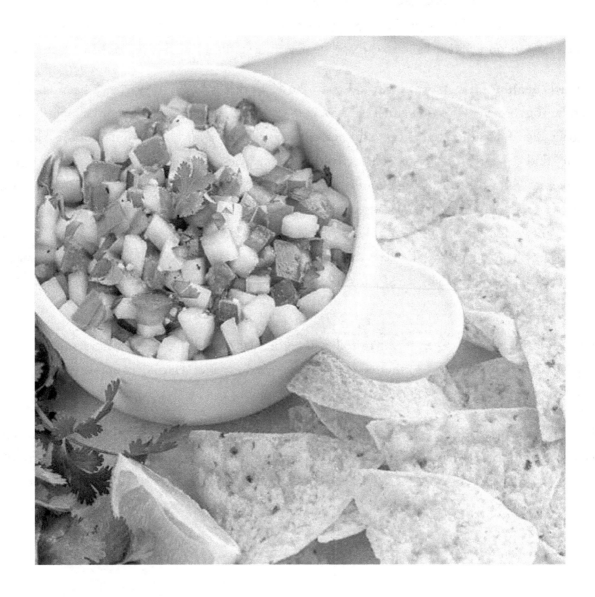

77. Perfect Cucumber Salsa

Preparation Time: 5 minutes

Cooking Time: 5 minutes

Servings: 10

Ingredients:

- 2 ½ cups cucumbers, peeled, seeded, and chopped
- 2 tsp. fresh cilantro, chopped
- 2 tsp. fresh parsley, chopped
- 1 ½ tbsp. fresh lemon juice
- 1 garlic clove, minced
- 1 small onion, chopped
- 2 large jalapeno peppers, chopped
- 1 ½ cups tomatoes, chopped
- ½ tsp. salt

Kitchen Equipment:

- Mixing bowl

Directions:

1. Mix all ingredients into the large mixing bowl until well combined.
2. Serve and enjoy.

Nutrition:

- 14 calories
- 0.2g fat
- 0.6g protein

77. Eggplant Chips

Preparation Time: 10 minutes

Cooking Time: 20 minutes

Servings: 15

Ingredients:

- 1 large eggplant, thinly sliced
- ¼ cup Parmesan cheese, grated
- 1 tsp. dried oregano
- ¼ tsp. dried basil
- ½ tsp. garlic powder
- ¼ cup olive oil
- ¼ tsp. pepper
- ½ tsp. salt

Kitchen Equipment:

- Oven
- Small bowl

Directions:

1. Preheat the oven to 325 F. In a small bowl, mix together oil and dried spices. Coat eggplant with oil and spice mixture and arrange eggplant slices on a baking tray.
2. Bake in a preheated oven for 15-20 minutes. Turn halfway through. Take it out from the oven and sprinkle with grated cheese. Serve and enjoy.

Nutrition:

- 77 calories 5.8g fat
- 3.5g protein

78. Lemon Chicken

Preparation Time: 10 minutes

Cooking Time: 45 minutes

Servings: 8

Ingredients:

- 8 chicken breasts, skinless and boneless
- 1/4 cup fresh lemon juice
- 2 tbsp. green onion, chopped
- 1 tbsp. oregano leaves

- 3 oz. feta cheese, crumbled
- 1/4 tsp. pepper

Kitchen Equipment:

- Oven
- Baking dish

Directions:

1. Prepare the oven to 350 F. Spray baking dish with cooking spray. Place chicken breasts in prepared baking dish. Drizzle with 2 tbsp. lemon juice and sprinkle with 1/2 tbsp. oregano and pepper.

2. Top with green onion and crumbled cheese. Drizzle with remaining lemon juice and oregano. Bake for 45 minutes. Serve and enjoy.

Nutrition:

- 245 calories
- 10.8g fat
- 34g protein

79. Spinach Meatballs

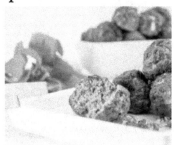

Preparation Time: 20 minutes

Cooking Time: 30 minutes

Servings: 4

Ingredients:

- 1 cup spinach, chopped
- 1 ½ lb. ground turkey breast
- 1 onion, chopped

- 3 cloves garlic, minced
- 1 egg, beaten
- ¼ cup milk
- ¾ cup breadcrumbs
- ½ cup Parmesan cheese, grated
- Salt and pepper to taste
- 2 tbsp. butter
- 2 tbsp. Keto flour
- 10 oz. Italian cheese, shredded
- ½ tsp. nutmeg, freshly grated
- ¼ cup parsley, chopped

Kitchen Equipment:

- Oven

Directions:

1. Set the oven at 400 F. Mix all the ingredients in a large bowl. Form meatballs from the mixture. Bake in the oven for 20 minutes.

Nutrition:

- 374 calories 18.5g fat 34.2g protein

80. Low Carb Beef Stir Fry

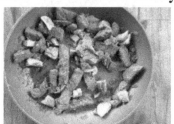

Preparation Time: 10 minutes

Cooking Time: 25 minutes

Servings: 3

Ingredients:

- ½ cup zucchini, spiral them into noodles about 6-inches each

- ¼ cup organic broccoli florets

- 1 bunch baby book choy, stem chopped

- 2 tbsp. avocado oil

- 2 tsp. coconut amines

- 1 small know of ginger, peeled, and cut

- 8 oz. skirt steak, thinly sliced into strips

Kitchen Equipment:

- Pan

Directions:

1. Heat the pan and add 1 tbsp. oil. Sear the steak on it on high heat. This should only take around 2 minutes per side.

2. Reduce the heat to medium and put in the broccoli, ginger, ghee, and coconut amines. Cook for a minute, stirring as often as possible.

3. Add in the book choy and cook for another minute

4. Finally, put the zucchini into the mix and cook. Note that zucchini noodles cook quickly, so you would want to pay close attention to this.

Nutrition:

- 104 calories 6g fat 31g protein

81. Crispy Peanut Tofu and Cauliflower Rice Stir-Fry

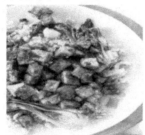

Preparation Time: 10 minutes

Cooking Time: 80 minutes

Servings: 4

Ingredients:

- 12 oz. tofu, extra-firm

- 1 tbsp. toasted sesame oil

- 2 cloves minced garlic

- 1 small cauliflower head

- For the sauce:

- 1 ½ tbsp. toasted sesame oil

- ½ tsp. chili garlic sauce

- 2 ½ tbsp. peanut butter

- ¼ cup low sodium soy sauce

- ½ cup light brown sugar

Kitchen Equipment:

- Oven

- Skillet

Directions:

1. Start by draining the tofu for 90 minutes before getting the meal ready. You can dry the tofu quickly by rolling it on an absorbent towel and putting something heavy on top. This will create a gentle pressure on the tofu to drain out the water.

2. Preheat the oven to 400 F. While the oven heats up, cube the tofu and prepare your baking sheet.

3. Bake for 25 minutes and allow it to cool.

4. Combine the sauce ingredients and whisk it thoroughly until you get that well-blended texture. You can add more ingredients, depending on your personal preferences with taste.

5. Put the tofu in the sauce and stir it quickly to coat the tofu thoroughly. Leave

it there for 15 minutes or more for a thorough marinate.

6. While the tofu marinates, shred the cauliflower into rice- size bits. You can also try buying cauliflower rice from the store to save yourself this step. Use fine grater or a food processor if ricing it manually.

7. Place skillet over medium heat. Start cooking the veggies on a bit of sesame oil and just a little bit of soy sauce. Set it aside.

8. Grab the tofu and put it on the pan. Stir the tofu frequently until it gets that nice golden-brown color. Do not worry if some of the tofu sticks to the pan – it will do that sometimes. Set aside.

9. Steam your cauliflower rice for 5 to 8 minutes. Add some sauce and stir thoroughly.

10. Now it is time to add up the ingredients together. Put the cauliflower rice with the veggies and tofu. Serve and enjoy. You can reheat this if there are leftovers but try not to leave it in the fridge for long.

Nutrition:

- 107 calories 9g fat 30g protein

82. Baked Lamb Ribs Macadamia with Tomato Salsa

Preparation Time: 10 minutes

Cooking Time: 45 minutes

Servings: 5

Ingredients:

- ½ lb. of fresh lamb ribs
- ½ cup of cherry tomatoes
- ½ tsp. pepper

- ½ cup of macadamia
- ½ tbsp. macadamia oil
- ¼ cup fresh parsley
- 1 tsp. balsamic vinegar
- 1 tsp. minced garlic
- 2 tbsp. extra virgin olive oil

Kitchen Equipment:

- Oven
- Aluminum foil
- Food processor

Directions:

1. Cut up the lamb ribs into strips or pieces

2. Preheat your oven to 204°C. Ensure that your baking tray is lined with aluminum foil.

3. Place the macadamia, garlic, parsley, pepper, and olive oil, in the food processor. Blend till the mixture is smooth and lump-free.

4. Rub your processed mixture all over your cut lamb pieces. Ensure that it is coated well enough.

5. Arrange your strips nicely in the baking tray and bake for 20-25 minutes.

6. While the lamb bakes, cut the cherry in pieces. You can cut each into four then place them in an aluminum cup.

7. Pour macadamia oil on the tomatoes. Use spoon to mix the oil and tomatoes without squishing it. The aim is to get the oil all over it. Take out your lamp and place on a plate. Place your tomatoes in the oven for 4-5 minutes.

8. Take out the tomatoes and pour sparse amounts of balsamic vinegar and stir. Pour the tomatoes on the lamb and serve warm.

Nutrition:

- 98 calories 7g fat 29g protein

83. Enticing Chicken and Broccoli Casserole

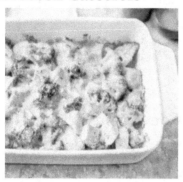

Preparation Time: 10 minutes

Cooking Time: 65 minutes

Servings: 4

Ingredients:

- 1 lb. broccoli florets
- 3 boneless, skinless chicken breasts
- 3 cups cheddar cheese, shredded or finely grated
- 1 cup of homemade zero-sugar mayonnaise
- 2 tbsp. coconut oil, melted
- ½ tsp. freshly cracked black pepper
- 1/3 cup homemade low-sodium chicken stock
- ½ tsp. sea salt
- 2 tbsp. freshly squeezed lemon juice

Kitchen Equipment:

- Oven
- Baking dish
- Aluminum foil

Directions:

1. Preheat your oven to 350 F. Brush baking dish with the coconut oil. Place the chicken pieces to the bottom of the baking dish. Spread the broccoli florets on top of the chicken. Spread half of the shredded cheddar cheese over the broccoli.

2. In a bowl, add the mayonnaise, chicken stock, sea salt, freshly cracked black pepper, and lemon juice. Pour this mixture over the chicken.

3. Sprinkle the remaining cheddar cheese over the baking dish and tightly cover the aluminum foil. Place the baking dish inside your oven and bake for 30 minutes.

4. Once done, remove the baking dish from your oven and carefully remove the aluminum foil. Return the baking dish to your oven and bake for 20 minutes. Serve and enjoy!

Nutrition:

- 107 calories
- 6g fat
- 28g protein

84. Sausage and Cheese Dip

Preparation Time: 10 minutes

Cooking Time: 80 minutes

Servings: 28

Ingredients:

- 8 oz cream cheese
- A pinch of salt and black pepper
- 16 oz sour cream
- 8 oz pepper jack cheese, chopped
- 15 oz canned tomatoes mixed with habaneros

- 1 lb. Italian sausage, ground
- ¼ cup green onions, chopped

Kitchen Equipment:

- Pan

Directions:

1. Preheat pan over medium heat, stir in sausage, and cook until it browns. Add tomatoes mix, stir and cook for 4 minutes more.

2. Season it and mix the green onions, stir and cook for 4 minutes. Spread pepper jack cheese on the bottom of your slow cooker.

3. Add cream cheese, sausage mix and sour cream, cover and cook on High for 2 hours. Uncover your slow cooker, stir dip, transfer to a bowl and serve. Enjoy!

Nutrition:

- 132 calories
- 6.79g protein
- 9.58g fat

85. Alfalfa Sprouts Salad

Preparation Time: 10 minutes

Cooking Time: 10 minutes

Servings: 4

Ingredients:

- 1 ½ tsp. Dark sesame oil
- 4 cups Alfalfa sprouts
- Salt and ground black pepper to taste
- 1 ½ tsp. Grapeseed oil
- ¼ cup Coconut yogurt

Kitchen Equipment:

- Bowl

Directions:

1. In a bowl, mix sprouts with yogurt, grape seed oil, sesame oil, salt, and pepper. Toss to coat and serve.

Nutrition:

- 83 calories
- 7.6g fat
- 1.6g protein

86. Convenient Tilapia Casserole

Preparation Time: 15 minutes

Cooking Time: 14 minutes

Servings: 4

Ingredients:

- 2 (14-oz.) cans sugar-free diced tomatoes with basil and garlic with juice
- 1/3 C. fresh parsley, chopped and divided
- ¼ tsp. dried oregano
- ½ tsp. red pepper flakes, crushed
- 4 (6-oz.) tilapia fillets
- 2 tbsp. fresh lemon juice
- 2/3 C. feta cheese, crumbled

Kitchen Equipment:

- Oven
- Shallow baking dish

Directions:

1. Preheat the oven to 4000 F. In a baking dish, stir in the tomatoes, ¼ C. of the parsley, oregano and red pepper flakes and mix until well combined.

2. Arrange the tilapia fillets over the tomato mixture in a single layer and drizzle with the lemon juice.

3. Place some tomato mixture over the tilapia fillets and sprinkle with the feta cheese evenly. Bake for about 12-14 minutes. Serve hot with the garnishing of remaining parsley.

Nutrition:

- 246 calories 9.4g Carbohydrates
- 37.2g protein

87. Quick Dinner Tilapia

Preparation Time: 15 minutes

Cooking Time: 6 minutes

Servings: 5

Ingredients:

- 2 tbsp. coconut oil
- 5 (5-oz.) tilapia fillets
- 2 tbsp. unsweetened coconut, shredded
- 3 garlic cloves, minced
- 1 tbsp. fresh ginger, minced
- 2 tbsp. low-sodium soy sauce
- 8 scallions, chopped

Kitchen Equipment:

- Large skillet

Directions:

1. In a large skillet, cook the coconut oil over medium heat and cook the tilapia fillets for about 2 minutes. Flip the side and stir in the coconut, garlic and ginger.

2. Cook for about 1 minute. Add the soy sauce and cook for about 1 minute. Add the scallions and cook for about 1-2 more minutes. Remove from heat and serve hot.

Nutrition:

- 189 calories

- 4.4g carbohydrates
- 27.7g protein

88. Stuffed Pepper Soup

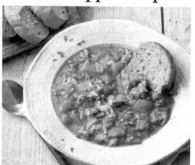

Preparation Time: 10 minutes

Cooking Time: 35 minutes

Servings: 6

Ingredients:

- 1 lb. ground beef
- 2 tbsp. coconut oil
- 1 small onion, finely chopped
- 2 large red bell peppers, seeds removed and chopped
- 1 (28-ounce) can diced tomatoes
- (14.5-ounce) can of tomato sauce
- 2 cups of homemade low-sodium chicken stock
- 2 cups of cauliflower rice
- 1 tsp. garlic powder
- 1 tsp. fine sea salt
- 1 tsp. freshly cracked black pepper

Kitchen Equipment:

- Instant pot

Directions:

1. Press the "Sauté" function on your Instant Pot and add the coconut oil, ground beef, bell peppers, and onions. Cook until the meat has browned and vegetables have softened, stirring frequently.

2. Add the remaining ingredients and stir until well combined. Close the lid and cook at high pressure for 15 minutes. When done, release the pressure and slowly take off the lid.

3. Stir the soup again and adjust the seasoning if necessary. Serve and enjoy!

Nutrition:

- 304 calories

- 10g fat

- 38g protein

89. Chicken Avocado Soup

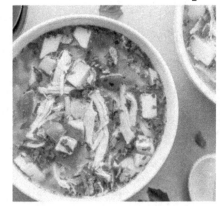

Preparation Time: 10 minutes

Cooking Time: 20 minutes

Servings: 4

Ingredients:

- 2 lb.s of boneless, skinless chicken thighs

- 1 green onion, finely chopped

- 1 jalapeno pepper, seeds remove and chopped

- 4 cups of homemade low-sodium chicken stock

- 2 tbsp. extra-virgin olive oil

- 6 garlic cloves, peeled and minced

- 2 tsp. ground cumin

- ½ cup of fresh cilantro, chopped

- 2 limes, freshly squeezed juice

- large avocados, pitted, peeled and mashed

Kitchen Equipment:

- Instant pot

Directions:

1. Press the "Sauté" setting on your Instant Pot and add the olive oil. Once hot, place the chicken thighs and sear for 4 minutes per side or until brown.

2. Add in the remaining ingredients except for heavy cream and avocados. Close the lid and cook at high pressure for 8 minutes. When the cooking is done, quickly release the tension and remove the cover. Place the chicken in a cutting board and shred using two forks.

3. Use an immersion blender to blend inside your Instant Pot. Stir in the mashed avocados, heavy cream, and shredded chicken. Serve and enjoy!

Nutrition:

- 317 calories

- 18g fat

- 37g protein

90. Hot Avocado Curry with Shrimp

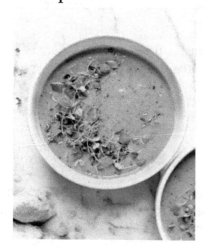

Preparation Time: 10 minutes

Cooking Time: 20 minutes

Servings: 2

Ingredients:

- ½ lb. of shrimp, peeled and deveined
- 2 cups of homemade low-sodium chicken stock
- 1 can(14-oz) coconut milk
- avocados, ripe, pitted, peeled and cut into quarters
- ½ tsp. cayenne pepper
- 1 tsp. fine sea salt
- 1 tbsp. freshly squeezed lime juice

Kitchen Equipment:

- Blender

Directions:

1. In a blender, add all the ingredients except for the shrimp. Blend until smooth and creamy. Pour in the mixture inside your Instant Pot along with the shrimp.

2. Close the lid. Cook at high pressure for 3 minutes. Then quickly release the tension

and remove the cover. Adjust the seasoning if necessary. Serve and enjoy!

Nutrition:

- 317 calories
- 12g fat
- 38g protein

91. Cream of Red Bell Pepper Soup

Preparation Time: 10 minutes

Cooking Time: 30 minutes

Servings: 4

Ingredients:

- 2 ½ lb.s of red bell peppers
- 4 tbsp. coconut oil, melted
- 2 shallots, finely chopped
- medium garlic cloves, peeled and minced
- cups of homemade low-sodium vegetable stock
- 2 tsp. red wine vinegar
- ½ tsp. cayenne pepper
- 1 tsp. fine sea salt
- 1 tsp. freshly cracked black pepper
- ½ cup of heavy cream

Kitchen Equipment:

- Instant pot

Directions:

1. Select the "Sauté" function on Instant Pot and pour the coconut oil. Once hot, stir in the bell peppers, shallots, and garlic cloves. Sauté until softened, stirring occasionally.

2. Add the remaining ingredients except for the heavy cream.

3. Close the lid and set at high pressure for at least 3 minutes. Once done, let it quickly release the tension and carefully remove the cover. Use an immersion blender to blend the soup until smooth. Stir in the heavy cream and adjust the seasoning if necessary.

4. Serve and enjoy!

Nutrition:

- 302 calories 12g fat 39g protein

92. King-Style Roasted Bell Pepper Soup

Preparation Time: 10 minutes

Cooking Time: 25 minutes

Servings: 3

Ingredients:

- 4 red bell peppers, chopped
- 4 tbsp. olive oil
- 4 garlic cloves, minced
- 1 large red onion, chopped
- ¼ cup of finely grated Parmesan cheese
- 2 celery stalks, chopped
- 4 cups of homemade low-sodium vegetable broth
- 1 tsp. freshly cracked black pepper
- 1 cup of heavy cream
- 1 tsp. sea salt

Kitchen Equipment:

- Oven
- Large bowl

Directions:

1. Preheat your oven to 400 F. In a large bowl, add the chopped red bell peppers with 2 tbsp. olive oil. Stir until well coated together.

2. Transfer the red bell peppers to a baking sheet and place it inside your oven.

3. Bake the red bell peppers inside your oven for 8 to 10 minutes. Slowly remove from the oven. Set aside. Cook the remaining 2 tbsp. olive oil in a large pot over medium-high heat.

4. Once hot, add the onion, garlic, and celery. Sauté for 8 minutes, stirring occasionally.

5. Add roasted red bell peppers and chicken stock. Bring to boil. Close the lid and reduce the heat to simmer. Puree soup using immersion blender. Season it well. Mix in the heavy cream and let it boil. Then, remove from the heat. Serve and sprinkle with Parmesan cheese.

Nutrition:

- 317 calories 14g fat
- 37g protein

93.Duck and Eggplant Casserole

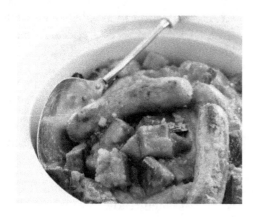

Preparation Time: 10 minutes

Cooking Time: 45 minutes

Servings: 4

Ingredients:

- 1-lb. ground duck meat
- 1 ½ tbsp. ghee, melted
- 1/3 cup double cream
- 1/2-lb. eggplant, peeled and sliced
- 1 ½ cups almond flour
- Salt and black pepper, to taste
- 1/2 tsp. fennel seeds
- 1/2 tsp. oregano, dried
- 8 eggs

Kitchen Equipment:

- Pie pan
- Oven

Directions:

1. Mix the almond flour with salt, black, fennel seeds, and oregano. Fold in one egg and the melted ghee and whisk to combine well.

2. Press the crust into the bottom of a lightly-oiled pie pan. Cook the ground duck until no longer pink for about 3 minutes, stirring continuously.

3. Whisk the remaining eggs and double cream. Fold in the browned meat and stir until everything is well incorporated. Pour the mixture into the prepared crust. Top with the eggplant slices.

4. Bake for about 40 minutes. Cut into four pieces.

Nutrition:

317 calories 10g fat

36g protein

94. Roasted Salmon Salad with Sesame Oil

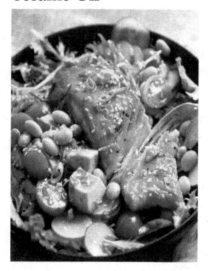

Preparation Time: 10 minutes

Cooking Time: 20 minutes

Servings: 6

Ingredients:

Salad:

- 1 medium lettuce, minced
- 1 medium red pepper, minced
- 1 medium yellow pepper, minced
- 2 large pieces (350 grams each) salmon fillet
- 4 tbsp. olive oil
- 2 tbsp. coconut amino acids
- 1 tsp. sesame oil
- ¼ cup green onions, chopped

Refueling:

- 4 tbsp. olive oil
- 5 tbsp. coconut amino acids
- 1 tsp. sesame oil

Kitchen Equipment:

- Skillet

Directions:

1. Cook ¾ olive oil in a skillet over medium heat. Add sesame oil, coconut oil, and liquid amino acids.

2. Chop the salmon into smaller pieces if necessary. Place the salmon slices in the skillet and cook for 5-7 minutes.

3. Turnover, continue cooking for another 5 minutes.

4. The pieces should be light pink to white when cut when ready.

5. While the salmon is cooking, put the lettuce and bell peppers in a salad bowl.

6. Prepare salad dressing in a smaller bowl. Once the salmon is done, place it on top of the lettuce and pepper leaves, add the dressing, stir the salad and enjoy!

Nutrition:

- 383 calories
- 27.14g fat
- 24.3g protein

95. Low Carb Chicken Salad with Chimichurri Sauce

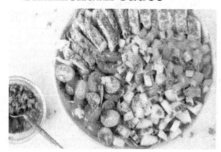

Preparation Time: 10 minutes

Cooking Time: 15 minutes

Servings: 5

Ingredients:

- 250 grams of various lettuce leaves
- 2 medium chicken breasts
- 2 medium avocados, diced
- ¼ cup olive oil
- 3 tbsp. red wine vinegar
- ¼ cup parsley, chopped
- 1 tbsp. oregano
- 1 tsp. chili pepper
- 1 tsp. garlic, minced

Kitchen Equipment:

- Non-stick skillet

Directions:

1. Preheat the non-stick skillet. Place the lettuce and diced avocado in a salad bowl. Cook the chicken breasts, fry them until white. Let the chicken cool.

2. In a small bowl, combine olive oil, vinegar, parsley, oregano, garlic, and chili. Cut the chicken breast into cubes. Add the chopped chicken fillet to the salad

and season with the classic chimichurri sauce.

3. Garnish the salad with additional chimichurri sauce and serve.

Nutrition:

- 285.94 calories
- 21.24 g fat — 17.24 g protein.

96. Potluck Lamb Salad

Preparation Time: 20 minutes

Cooking Time: 10 minutes

Servings: 4

Ingredients:

- 2 tbsp. olive oil, divided
- 12 oz. grass-fed lamb leg steaks, trimmed
- Salt and black pepper, to taste
- 6½ oz. halloumi cheese, cut into thick slices
- 2 jarred roasted red bell peppers, sliced thinly
- 2 cucumbers, cut into thin ribbons
- 3 C. fresh baby spinach
- 2 tbsp. balsamic vinegar

Kitchen Equipment:

- Skillet

Directions:

1. In a skillet, heat 1 tbsp. the oil over medium-high heat and cook the lamb steaks for about 4-5 minutes per side or until desired doneness.

2. Transfer the lamb steaks onto a cutting board for about 5 minutes.

3. Then cut the lamb steaks into thin slices. In the same skillet, add halloumi and

cook for about 1-2 minutes per side or until golden.

4. In a salad bowl, add the lamb, halloumi, bell pepper, cucumber, salad leaves, vinegar, and remaining oil and toss to combine.

5. Serve immediately.

Nutrition:

- 420 calories

- 35.4g protein — 1.3g fiber.

asparagus well. In a serving bowl, add the asparagus and remaining salad ingredients and mix.

2. In another bowl, add all the dressing ingredients and beat until well combined. Place the dressing over salad and gently toss to coat well. Serve immediately.

Nutrition:

- 223 calories

- 8.5g Carbohydrates — 3.5g fiber.

97. Spring Supper Salad

Preparation Time: 15 minutes

Cooking Time: 5 minutes

Servings: 5

Ingredients:

For Salad:

- 1 lb. fresh asparagus

- ½ lb. smoked salmon, cut into bite-sized pieces

- 2 heads red leaf lettuce, torn

- ¼ C. pecans, toasted and chopped

For Dressing:

- ¼ C. olive oil

- 2 tbsp. fresh lemon juice

- 1 tsp. Dijon mustard

- Salt and black pepper, to taste

Kitchen Equipment:

- Pan

Directions:

1. In a boiling water, stir in the asparagus and cook for about 5 minutes. Drain the

98. Chicken-of-Sea Salad

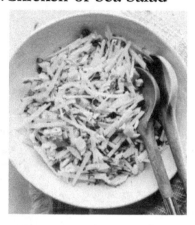

Preparation Time: 15 minutes

Cooking Time: 5 minutes

Servings: 6

Ingredients:

- 2 (6-oz.) cans olive oil-packed tuna, drained
- 2 (6-oz.) cans water packed tuna, drained
- ¾ C. mayonnaise
- 2 celery stalks, chopped
- ¼ of onion, chopped
- 1 tbsp. fresh lime juice
- 2 tbsp. mustard
- Freshly ground black pepper, to taste
- 6 C. fresh baby arugula

Kitchen Equipment:

- Large bowl

Directions:

1. In a large bowl, incorporate all the ingredients except arugula and gently stir to combine. Divide arugula onto serving plates and top with tuna mixture. Serve immediately.

Nutrition:

- 325 calories 27.4g protein
- 1.1g fiber

99. Keto Kohlrabi Salad

Preparation Time: 10 minutes

Cooking Time: 0 minute

Servings: 2

Ingredients:

- 450g kohlrabi
- 225ml plain mayonnaise or vegan mayonnaise
- Salt and pepper
- Fresh parsley (optional)

Kitchen Equipment:

- Bowl

Directions:

1. Clean the kohlrabi. Be sure to cut out any tough parts of the cabbage. Slice, chop, or chop and place in a bowl. Add mayonnaise to the cabbage and, if desired, fresh herbs. Season the kohlrabi salad with salt and pepper to taste.

Nutrition:

- 4g fiber 41g fat
- 405 calories

100. Coconut Cake

Preparation Time: 10 minutes

Cooking Time: 20 minutes

Servings: 8

Ingredients: parated

- ½ tsp. baking powder
- 5 eggs, se
- ½ tsp. vanilla
- ½ cup butter softened
- ½ cup erythritol
- ¼ cup unsweetened coconut milk
- ½ cup coconut flour
- Pinch of salt

Kitchen Equipment:

- Oven
- Cake pan

Directions:

1. Start to preheat oven to 400 F/ 200 C. Grease cake pan with butter and set aside. In a bowl, beat sweetener and butter until combined. Add egg yolks, coconut milk, and vanilla and mix well.

2. Add baking powder, coconut flour, and salt and stir well. In another bowl, beat egg whites until stiff peak forms. Combine the egg whites into the cake mixture.

3. Pour batter in a prepared cake pan and bake in preheated oven for 20 minutes. Slice and serve.

152. Grilled Whole Chicken

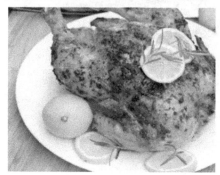

Preparation Time: 20 minutes

Cooking Time: 20 minutes

Servings: 6

Ingredients:

- ¼ cup butter, melted

- 2 tbsp. fresh lemon juice

- 2 tsp. fresh lemon zest, grated finely

- 1 tsp. dried oregano, crushed

- 2 tsp. paprika

- 1 tsp. onion powder

- 1 tsp. garlic powder

- Salt and ground black pepper, as required

- 1 (4 lb.) grass-fed whole chicken, neck and giblets removed

Kitchen Equipment:

- Grill

- Bowl

Directions:

1. Preheat the grill to medium heat. Grease the grill grate. In a bowl, add the butter, lemon juice, lemon zest, oregano, spices, salt, and black pepper, and mix until well combined. Place chicken onto a large cutting board, breast-side down.

2. With a sharp knife, cut along both sides of backbone and then remove the backbone. Now, flip the breast side of chicken up and open it like a book. Flatten the breast with your hands.

3. Coat the whole chicken with the oil mixture generously. Arrange the chicken onto the grill and cook for about 16–20 minutes, flipping once halfway through.

4. Remove from the grill and place the chicken onto a cutting board for about 5–10 minutes before carving.

5. Slice the chicken into desired-sized pieces and serve.

Nutrition:

- 532 calories 17g fat 0.5g fiber

152.Grilled Chicken Breast

Preparation Time: 15 minutes

Cooking Time: 14 minutes

Servings: 4

Ingredients:

- ¼ cup balsamic vinegar
- 2 tbsp. olive oil
- 1½ tsp. fresh lemon juice
- ½ tsp. lemon-pepper seasoning
- 4 (6 oz.) grass-fed boneless skinless chicken breast halves, lb.ed slightly

Kitchen Equipment:

- Glass baking dish
- Grill

Directions:

1. In a glass baking dish, place the vinegar, oil, lemon juice, and seasoning, and mix well. Add the chicken breasts and coat with the mixture generously. Refrigerate to marinate for about 25–30 minutes.

2. Preheat the grill to medium heat. Grease the grill grate. Remove the chicken from bowl and discard the remaining marinade. Move the chicken breasts onto the grill and cover with the lid.

3. Cook for about 5–7 minutes per side or until desired doneness. Serve hot.

Nutrition:

- 258 calories 11.3g fat
- 0.1g fiber

153.Glazed Chicken Thighs

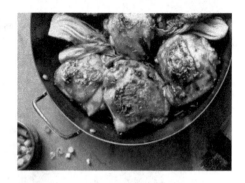

Preparation Time: 15 minutes

Cooking Time: 35 minutes

Servings: 8

Ingredients:

- ½ cup balsamic vinegar
- 1/3 cup low-sodium soy sauce
- 3 tbsp. Yukon syrup
- 4 tbsp. olive oil
- 3 tbsp. chili sauce
- 2 tbsp. garlic, minced
- Salt and ground black pepper, as required
- 8 (6 oz.) grass-fed skinless chicken thighs

Kitchen Equipment:

- Bowl
- Large plastic zipper bag
- Oven
- Small pan

Directions:

1. Combine all ingredients (except chicken thighs and sesame seeds) and beat them until well combined. In a large plastic zipper bag, add half of marinade and chicken thighs. Seal the bag and shake to coat well.

2. Pace the bag in refrigerator for at least 1 hour, turning bag twice. Reserve

remaining marinade in the refrigerator until using. Preheat your oven to 425°F.

3. In a small pan, add reserved marinade over medium heat and bring to a boil. Cook for about 3–5 minutes, stirring occasionally. Remove the pan of sauce from heat and set aside to cool slightly.

4. Pull out the chicken from the bag and discard excess marinade. Arrange chicken thighs into a 9x13-inch baking dish in a single layer and coat with some of the cooked marinade.

5. Bake for about 30 minutes, coating with the cooked marinade slightly after every 10 minutes. Serve hot.

Nutrition:

- 406 calories 19.6g fat 0.1g fiber

154.Bacon-Wrapped Chicken Breasts

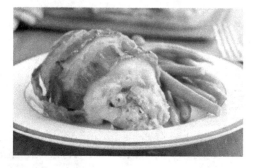

Preparation Time: 15 minutes

Cooking Time: 33 minutes

Servings: 4

Ingredients:

Chicken Marinade :

- 3 tbsp. balsamic vinegar
- 3 tbsp. olive oil
- 2 tbsp. water
- 1 garlic clove, minced

- 1 tsp. dried Italian seasoning
- ½ tsp. dried rosemary
- Salt and ground black pepper, as required
- 4 (6 oz.) grass-fed skinless, boneless chicken breasts

Stuffing:

- 16 fresh basil leaves
- 1 large fresh tomato, sliced thinly
- 4 provolone cheese slices
- 8 bacon slices
- ¼ cup Parmesan cheese, grated freshly

Kitchen Equipment:

- Bowl
- Oven

Directions:

1. *For marinade*: In a bowl, add all ingredients (except chicken) and mix until well combined.

2. Place 1 chicken breast onto a smooth surface. Hold a sharp knife parallel to work surface, slice the chicken breast horizontally, without cutting all the way through.

3. Repeat with the remaining chicken breasts. Place the breasts in the bowl of marinade and toss to coat well. Refrigerate, covered, for at least 30 minutes.

4. Preheat your oven to 500 F. Grease a baking dish. Remove the chicken breast from the bowl and arrange onto a smooth surface.

5. Place 4 basil leaves onto the bottom half of a chicken breast. Followed by 2–3 tomato slices and 1 provolone cheese slice. Now, fold the top half over the filling.

6. Wrap the breast with 3 bacon slices and secure with toothpicks. Repeat with the remaining chicken breasts and filling. Arrange breasts into the prepared baking dish in a single layer.

7. Bake for about 30 minutes, flipping one halfway through. Remove from the oven and sprinkle each chicken breast with Parmesan cheese evenly. Bake for about 2–3 minutes more. Serve hot.

Nutrition:

- 633 calories
- 36g fat
- 0.3g fiber

155. Chicken Parmigiana

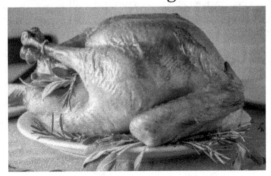

Preparation Time: 15 minutes

Cooking Time: 26 minutes

Servings: 5

Ingredients:

- 5 (6 oz.) grass-fed skinless, boneless chicken breasts
- 1 large organic egg, beaten
- ½ cup superfine blanched almond flour
- ¼ cup Parmesan cheese, grated
- ½ tsp. dried parsley
- ½ tsp. paprika
- ½ tsp. garlic powder
- Salt and ground black pepper, as required
- ¼ cup olive oil
- 1 cup sugar-free tomato sauce
- 5 oz. mozzarella cheese, thinly sliced
- 2 tbsp. fresh parsley, chopped

Kitchen Equipment:

- Oven
- Parchment paper
- Meat mallet
- Shallow dish

Directions:

1. Preheat your oven to 375 F. Arrange 1 chicken breast between 2 pieces of parchment paper. With a meat mallet, lb. the chicken breast into ½-inch thickness

2. Repeat with the remaining chicken breasts. Add the beaten egg into a shallow dish. Place the almond flour, Parmesan, parsley, spices, salt, and black pepper in another shallow dish, and mix well.

3. Dip chicken breasts into the whipped egg and then coat with the flour mixture. Heat the oil in a deep wok over medium-high heat and deep-fry the chicken breasts on each side.

4. With a slotted spoon, transfer the chicken breasts onto a paper towel-lined plate to drain. Pour about ½ cup of tomato sauce and spread evenly. Arrange the chicken breasts over marinara sauce in a single layer.

5. Top with the remaining tomato sauce, followed by mozzarella cheese slices. Bake for about 20 minutes or until done completely. Remove from the oven and serve hot with the garnishing of parsley.

Nutrition:

- 458 calories
- 25.4g fat
- 7.9g carbs

156. Roasted Turkey

Preparation Time: 15 minutes

Cooking Time: 80 minutes

Servings: 12

Ingredients:

Marinade:

- 1 (2-inch) piece fresh ginger, grated finely
- 3 large garlic cloves, crushed
- 1 green chili, chopped finely
- 2 tsp. ground turmeric
- 1 tsp. fresh lemon zest, grated finely
- 5 oz. plain Greek yogurt
- 3 tbsp. homemade tomato puree
- 2 tbsp. fresh lemon juice
- 1½ tbsp. garam masala
- 1 tbsp. ground cumin

Turkey:

- 1 (9 lb.) whole turkey
- Salt and ground black pepper, as required
- 1 garlic clove, halved
- 1 lime, halved
- 1 lemon, halved

Kitchen Equipment:

- Bowl
- Large baking dish
- Oven
- Aluminum foil

Directions:

1. *For marinade*: In a bowl, mix all ingredients. With a fork, pierce the turkey completely. In a large baking dish, place the turkey and rub with the marinade mixture evenly.

2. Refrigerate to marinate overnight. Remove the turkey from the refrigerator and set aside for about 30 minutes before cooking. Preheat your oven to 390 F.

3. Season the turkey evenly and stuff the cavity with garlic, lime, and lemon. Arrange the turkey in a large roasting pan and roast for about 30 minutes.

4. Lower the temperature of the oven to 350 F. Roast for about 3 hours. (If skin becomes brown during roasting, then cover with a piece of foil.) Remove from the oven and palace the turkey onto a platter for about 15–20 minutes before carving.

5. With a sharp knife, cut the turkey into desired-sized pieces and serve.

Nutrition:

- 595 calories
- 17.3g fat
- 2.3g carbs

157. Roasted Turkey Breast

Preparation Time: 15 minutes

Cooking Time: 75 minutes

Servings: 14

Ingredients:

- 1 tsp. onion powder
- ½ tsp. garlic powder
- Salt and ground black pepper, as required
- 1 (7-lb.) bone-in turkey breast

- 1½ cups Italian dressing

Kitchen Equipment:

- Oven
- 13x9 baking dish
- Bowl

Directions:

1. Preheat your oven to 325°F. Grease a 13x9-inch baking dish. In a bowl, add the onion powder, garlic powder, salt, and black pepper, and mix well.

2. Rub the turkey breast with the seasoning mixture generously. Arrange the turkey breast into the prepared baking dish and top with the Italian dressing evenly. Bake for about 2–2½ hours, coating with pan juices occasionally.

3. Remove from the oven and palace the turkey breast onto a platter for about 10–15 minutes before slicing. With a sharp knife, cut the turkey breast into desired-sized slices and serve.

Nutrition:

- 459 calories
- 2.8g carbs
- 23.3g fat

158.Meatloaf

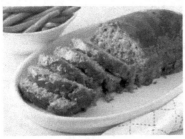

Preparation Time: 15 minutes

Cooking Time: 65 minutes

Servings: 8

Ingredients:

- 2 lb. lean ground pork
- ½ cup yellow onion, chopped
- ½ cup green bell pepper, seeded and chopped
- 2 garlic cloves, minced
- 1 cup cheddar cheese, grated
- ¼ cup sugar-free ketchup
- ¼ cup sugar-free HP steak sauce
- 2 organic eggs, beaten
- 1 tsp. dried thyme, crushed
- Salt and ground black pepper, as required
- 3 cups fresh spinach, chopped
- 2 cups mozzarella cheese, grated freshly

Kitchen Equipment:

- Oven
- Baking dish
- Large bowl

Directions:

1. Preheat your oven to 350 F. Lightly grease a baking dish. In a large bowl, add all the ingredients (except spinach and mozzarella cheese) and mix until well combined. Place a large wax paper onto a smooth surface. Place the meat mixture over wax paper. Add the spinach over meat mixture, pressing slightly.

2. Top with the mozzarella cheese. Roll the wax paper around meat mixture to form a meatloaf.

3. Carefully, remove the wax paper and place meatloaf onto the prepared baking dish. Bake for about 1-1¼ hours.

4. Remove the baking dish from the oven and set aside for about 10 minutes before serving. With a sharp knife, cut into desired-size slices and serve.

Nutrition:

- 280 calories 5.5g carbs 11.1g fat

159. Rosemary Beef Tenderloin

Preparation Time: 10 minutes

Cooking Time: 50 minutes

Servings: 10

Ingredients:

- 1 (3 lb.) grass-fed center-cut beef tenderloin roast
- 4 garlic cloves, minced
- 1 tbsp. fresh rosemary, minced and divided
- Salt and ground black pepper, as required
- 2 tbsp. olive oil

Kitchen Equipment:

- oven
- large shallow roasting pan

Directions:

1. Preheat your oven to 425 F. Grease a large shallow roasting pan. Place beef into the prepared roasting pan.

2. Rub the beef with garlic, rosemary, salt, and black pepper and drizzle with oil. Roast the beef for about 45–50 minutes. Remove from oven and place the roast onto a cutting board for about 10 minutes. With a sharp knife, cut beef tenderloin into desired-sized slices and serve.

Nutrition:

- 314 calories 0.4g carbs 16.9g fat

160. Garlicky Prime Rib Roast

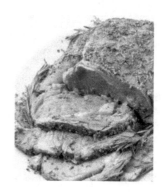

Preparation Time: 15 minutes

Cooking Time: 75 minutes

Servings: 15

Ingredients:

- 10 garlic cloves, minced
- 2 tsp. dried thyme, crushed
- 2 tbsp. olive oil
- Salt and ground black pepper, as required
- 1 (10 lb.) grass-fed prime rib roast

Kitchen Equipment:

- Bowl
- large roasting pan
- oven

Directions:

1. In a bowl, add the garlic, thyme, oil, salt, and black pepper, and mix until well combined. Coat the rib roast evenly with garlic mixture and arrange in a large roasting pan, fatty side up. Set aside to marinate at the room temperature for at least 1 hour.

2. Preheat your oven to 500 F. Place the roasting pan into the oven and roast for about 20 minutes. Now, reduce the temperature to 320 F and roast for about 65–75 minutes.

3. Remove from the oven and place the rib roast onto a cutting board for about 10–15 minutes before slicing. With a sharp

knife, cut the rib roast into desired-sized slices and serve.

Nutrition:

- 499 calories 0.6g carbs 0.1g fiber

161. Beef Wellington

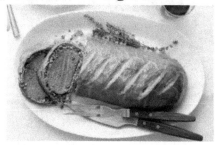

Preparation Time: 20 minutes

Cooking Time: 40 minutes

Servings: 4

Ingredients:

- 2 (4 oz.) grass-fed beef tenderloin steaks, halved
- Salt and ground black pepper, as required
- 1 tbsp. butter
- 1 cup mozzarella cheese, shredded
- ½ cup almond flour
- 4 tbsp. liver pate

Kitchen Equipment:

- Oven
- Baking sheet
- Frying pan
- Microwave
- Parchment paper

Directions:

1. Preheat your oven to 400 F. Grease a baking sheet. Season the steaks with salt and black pepper evenly.

2. In a frying pan, melt the butter over medium-high heat and sear the beef steaks for about 2–3 minutes per side. Remove frying pan from the heat and set aside to cool completely.

3. In a microwave-safe bowl, add the mozzarella cheese and microwave for about 1 minute. Remove from the microwave and immediately, stir in the almond flour until a dough form. Place the dough between 2 parchment paper pieces and with a rolling pin, roll to flatten it. Remove the upper parchment paper piece. Divide the rolled dough into 4 pieces.

4. Place 1 tbsp. pate onto each dough piece and top with 1 steak piece.

5. Cover each steak piece with dough completely. Arrange the covered steak pieces onto the prepared baking sheet in a single layer. Bake for about 20–30 minutes or until the pastry is a golden-brown. Serve warm.

Nutrition:

- 545 calories 36.6g fat 3g fiber

162. Beef with Mushroom Sauce

Preparation Time: 15 minutes

Cooking Time: 28 minutes

Servings: 4

Ingredients:

- Mushroom Sauce:
- 2 tbsp. butter
- 3 garlic cloves, minced
- 1 tsp. dried tyme
- 1½ cups fresh button mushrooms, sliced
- Salt and ground black pepper, as required
- 7 oz. cream cheese, softened
- ½ cup heavy cream

Steak:

- 4 (6 oz.) grass-fed beef tenderloin filets

- Salt and ground black pepper, as required
- 2 tbsp. butter

Kitchen Equipment:

- Saucepan
- Large cast-iron wok

Directions:

For mushroom sauce:

1. In a wok, melt butter over medium heat and sauté the garlic and thyme for about 1 minute.

2. Stir in the mushrooms, salt, and black pepper, and cook for about 5–7 minutes, stirring frequently. Now, adjust the heat to low and stir in cream cheese until smooth.

3. Stir in cream and cook for about 2–3 minutes or until heated completely.

4. Meanwhile, rub the beef filets evenly with salt and black pepper.

5. In a large cast-iron wok, melt the butter over medium heat and cook the filets for about 5–7 minutes per side. Remove the wok of mushroom gravy from heat and stir in the bacon.

6. Place the filets onto serving plates and serve with the topping of mushroom gravy.

Nutrition:

- 687 calories
- 60g fat
- 3.5g Total

163. Herbed Rack of Lamb

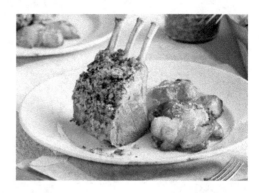

Preparation Time: 15 minutes

Cooking Time: 29 minutes

Servings: 8

Ingredients:

- 2 (2½ lb.) grass-fed racks of lamb, chine bones removed and trimmed
- Salt and ground black pepper, as required
- 2 tbsp. Dijon mustard
- 2 tsp. fresh rosemary, chopped
- 2 tsp. fresh parsley, chopped
- 2 tsp. fresh thyme, chopped

Kitchen Equipment:

- Charcoal grill
- Grill grate

Directions:

1. Preheat the charcoal grill to high heat. Grease the grill grate. Season the rack of lamb evenly with salt and black pepper. Coat the meaty sides of racks with mustard, followed by fresh herbs, pressing gently.

2. Carefully, push the coals to one side of the grill. Place racks of lamb over the coals, meaty side down and cook for about 6 minutes. Now, flip the racks and cook for about 3 more minutes.

3. Again, flip the racks down and move to the cooler side of the grill. Cover the grill and cook for about 20 minutes.

4. Remove from the grill and place racks of lamb onto a cutting board for about 10 minutes. With a sharp knife, carve the racks of lamb into chops and serve.

Nutrition:

- 532 calories 21g fat 0.4g fiber

164. Roasted Leg of Lamb

Preparation Time: 15 minutes

Cooking Time: 75 minutes

Servings: 8

Ingredients:

- 1/3 cup fresh parsley, minced
- 4 garlic cloves, minced
- 1 tsp. fresh lemon zest, finely grated
- 1 tbsp. ground coriander
- 1 tbsp. ground cumin
- 1 tbsp. smoked paprika
- 1 tbsp. red pepper flakes, finely crushed
- ½ tsp. ground allspice
- 1/3 cup olive oil
- 1 (5 lb.) grass-fed bone-in leg of lamb, trimmed

Kitchen Equipment:

- Large bowl
- Oven
- Roasting pan

Directions:

1. In a large bowl, place all ingredients (except the leg of lamb) and mix well.

2. Coat the leg of lamb with marinade mixture generously.

3. With a plastic wrap, cover the leg of lamb and refrigerate to marinate for about 6–8 hours.

4. Remove from the refrigerator and keep in room temperature for about 30 minutes before roasting.

5. Preheat your oven to 350 F. Arrange the oven rack in the center of oven.

6. Arrange a lightly, greased rack in the roasting pan.

7. Place the leg of lamb over rack into the roasting pan.

8. Roast for about 1¼-1½ hours, rotating the pan once halfway through.

9. Remove from the oven and place the leg of lamb onto a cutting board for about 10–15 minutes.

10. With a sharp knife, cut the leg of lamb into desired-size slices and serve.

Nutrition:

- 610 calories 29.6g fat 0.7g fiber

165.Stuffed Pork Tenderloin

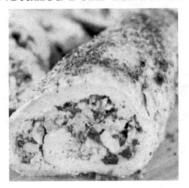

Preparation Time: 20 minutes

Cooking Time: 70 minutes

Servings: 3

Ingredients:

- 1 lb. pork tenderloin
- 1 tbsp. unsalted butter
- 2 tsp. garlic, minced
- 2 oz. fresh spinach
- 4 oz. cream cheese, softened
- 1 tsp. liquid smoke
- Salt and ground black pepper, as required

Kitchen Equipment:

- Oven
- Aluminum foil
- Casserole dish
- Meat tenderizer

Directions:

1. Preheat your oven to 350 F. Line a casserole dish with a piece of foil. Arrange the pork tenderloin between 2 plastic wraps and with a meat tenderizer, lb. until flat.

2. Carefully, cut the edges of tenderloin to shape into a rectangle. Melt the butter in a large wok over medium heat and sauté the garlic for about 1 minute.

3. Add the spinach, cream cheese, liquid smoke, salt, and black pepper, and cook for about 3–4 minutes. Remove the wok from heat and let it cool slightly.

4. Place the spinach mixture onto pork tenderloin about ½-inch from the edges.

5. Carefully, roll tenderloin into a log and secure with toothpicks. Arrange tenderloin into the prepared casserole dish, seam-side down.

6. Bake for about 1¼ hours. Remove the casserole dish from oven and let it cool slightly before cutting. Cut the tenderloin into desired-size slices and serve.

Nutrition:

- 389 calories 22.4g fat
- 2.3g carbs

166.Mini Parsnip Pancakes

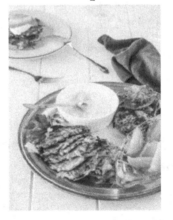

Preparation Time: 15 minutes

Cooking Time: 24 minutes

Servings: 4

Ingredients:

- 1 parsnip, finely grated
- 1 small white onion, finely grated
- ¼ tsp. nutmeg powder

- Salt and black pepper to taste
- 2 eggs
- 1 cup (227g) almond flour
- 1 cup (227g) grated cheddar cheese
- 4 tbsp. avocado oil for frying

Kitchen Equipment:

- Bowl
- Large skillet

Directions:

1. In a bowl, mix the parsnip, onions, nutmeg powder, salt, black pepper, eggs, almond flour, and Monterey Jack cheese until well-combined. Heat the avocado oil in a large skillet over medium heat.

2. Working in batches, use a scoop to add drops of the mixture into the skillet with intervals. Press down to form patties and fry each side until golden brown and compacted. Remove the pancakes to a paper towel-lined plate to drain grease and make more pancakes.

Nutrition:

- 784 calories
- 79.88g fat
- 1.7g fiber

167. Creamy Mashed Cauliflower

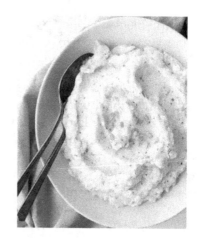

Preparation Time: 15 minutes

Cooking Time: 12 minutes

Servings: 4

Ingredients:

- 2 (236g) head cauliflowers, cut into florets
- 1 cup (227g) almond milk
- 1/3 cup (74g) heavy cream
- 4 garlic cloves, minced
- ¼ tsp. nutmeg powder
- Salt and black pepper to taste
- 4 tbsp. unsalted butter, room temperature
- 2 tbsp. cream cheese
- 1 tbsp. chopped fresh scallions

Kitchen Equipment:

- Pot

Directions:

1. Add the cauliflower and about 2 cups of salted water to a pot, cover, and bring to a boil over medium heat. Reduce the heat and simmer for 10 minutes or until the cauliflower is tender. Drain the cauliflower and pour it into a bowl.

2. Meanwhile as the cauliflower cooked, pour the almond milk in a pot and add the heavy cream, garlic, nutmeg powder,

salt, and black pepper. Warm over medium-low heat for 1 to 2 minutes, but don't let boil.

3. Mash the cauliflower using a masher until smooth. Add the butter, cream cheese, and pour the warm almond milk mixture. Mix well until the butter and cream cheese melt and combine well with the other ingredients. Garnish with the scallions and serve warm.

Nutrition:

- 662 calories

- 72.08g fat 5.02g carbs

168. Korean Braised Turnips

Preparation Time: 15 minutes

Cooking Time: 27 minutes

Servings: 4

Ingredients:

- 1 large turnip, peeled and cubed

- 2 tbsp. almond oil

- 2 garlic cloves, minced

- 6 tbsp. Coconut aminos

- 3 tbsp. Swerve brown sugar

- ½ cup (125ml) vegetable broth

- 1 cup grated Gruyere cheese

Kitchen Equipment:

- Deep skillet

Directions:

1. Add the turnip to a pot and cover with slightly salted water. Boil over medium heat for 5 minutes or slightly tender. Drain the turnips.

2. Heat the almond oil in a deep skillet and sauté the garlic until fragrant, 30 seconds.

3. In a bowl, mix the Coconut aminos and Swerve brown sugar.

4. Toss the turnips in the peanut oil and pour on the Coconut aminos mixture. Sauté for 1 minute and add the vegetable broth. Stir well and cook for 20 minutes or until the turnips soften and the liquid reduces.

5. Spoon the turnips onto serving plates, top with the Gruyere cheese and garnish with the peanuts.

Nutrition:

- 182 calories

- 15.57g fat

- 0.6g fiber

169. Garlic Sautéed Rapini

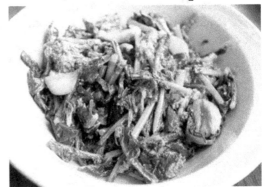

Preparation Time: 10 minutes

Cooking Time: 11 minutes

Servings: 4

Ingredients:

- 2 tbsp. avocado oil

- 4 garlic cloves, minced

- 2 cups (454 g) rapini

- Salt to taste

- 1 cup (227 g) grated Monterey Jack cheese for topping

- 2 tbsp. toasted almond flakes for topping

-

Kitchen Equipment:

- Large skillet

Directions:

1. Heat the avocado oil in a large skillet and sauté the garlic until fragrant, 30 seconds. Mix in the rapini and cook for 8 to 10 minutes or until tender. Season with salt.

2. Dish the rapini onto serving plates, top with the Monterrey Jack cheese, almonds, and serve immediately.

Nutrition:

- 254 calories 23.91g fat 0.6g fiber

170.Broccoli Fried Cheese

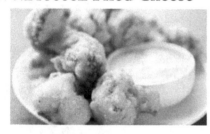

Preparation Time: 15 minutes

Cooking Time: 14 minutes

Servings: 4

Ingredients:

- 1 (225g) head broccoli, cut into florets
- 2 eggs
- 1 cup (227g) grated cheddar cheese
- 1/3 cup (74g) grated Monterrey Jack cheese
- 2 tbsp. butter

Kitchen Equipment:

- Steamer – Bowl - Large skillet

Directions:

1. Add the broccoli to a steamer and cook for 10 minutes or until tender. Pour the broccoli into a bowl and let cool. Crack on the eggs and mix with the cheeses.

2. Working the batches, melt the butter in a large skillet and fry the broccoli on both sides until golden brown. Remove the broccoli to a plate and serve warm.

Nutrition:

- 240 calories 20.75g fat 0.3g fiber

171.Spicy Butter Baked Asparagus

Preparation Time: 15 minutes

Cooking Time: 15 minutes

Servings: 4

Ingredients:

- ½ lb. (227g) asparagus, hard stems removed
- ½ cup (113g) salted butter, melted
- 1 tsp. cayenne pepper
- Salt and black pepper to taste
- 1 cup grated Monterrey Jack cheese for topping

Kitchen Equipment:

- Oven - Baking tray

Directions:

1. Preheat the oven to 425 F/220 C. Spread the asparagus on a baking tray. In a small bowl, mix the butter, cayenne pepper, salt, and black pepper. Drizzle the mixture on the asparagus and toss well with a spatula. Scatter the Monterrey Jack cheese on top.

2. Bake in the oven for 15 minutes or until golden brown and the asparagus are tender. Serve afterwards.

Nutrition:

- 253 calories 24.01g fat 1.3g fiber

172. Grilled Zucchini with Pecan Gremolata

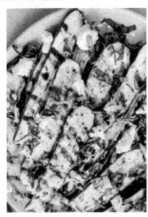

Preparation Time: 45 minutes

Cooking Time: 8 minutes

Servings: 4

Ingredients:

- 2 zucchinis, cut into strips
- Salt and black pepper to taste
- 4 tbsp. sugar-free maple syrup
- ½ cup (113g) olive oil, divided
- 2 scallions, chopped
- 8 garlic cloves, minced
- 1 cup (227g) toasted pecans, chopped
- 8 tbsp. pork rinds
- 2 tbsp. chopped fresh parsley
- 1 tbsp. plain vinegar

Kitchen Equipment:

- Grill pan
- Bowl

Directions:

1. Sprinkle the zucchinis with salt and let sit for 15 to 30 minutes to release liquid. After, pat dry with a paper towel. In a bowl, mix 2 tbsp. olive oil with the maple syrup and toss with the zucchinis.

2. Heat a grill pan over medium heat and grill the zucchinis on both sides until golden brown. Remove onto a serving platter.

3. In a bowl, mix the remaining olive oil, scallions, garlic, pecans, pork rinds, parsley, and vinegar. Spoon the gremolata all over the zucchinis and enjoy!

Nutrition:

- 1852 calories
- 184.1g fat
- 1.4g fiber

173. Coconut Cauli Fried Rice

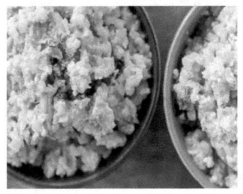

Preparation Time: 10 minutes

Cooking Time: 8 minutes

Servings: 4

Ingredients:

- 2 tbsp. coconut oil
- 1 small red bell pepper, deseeded and chopped
- 1 scallion, chopped + extra for garnish

- 2 garlic cloves, minced
- 4 eggs, beaten
- 1 cup (227g) cauliflower rice
- 1 tbsp. Coconut aminos
- Salt and black pepper to taste
- 1 cup grated cheddar cheese

Kitchen Equipment:

- Wok

Directions:

1. Melt the coconut oil in wok and stir-fry the bell peppers for 5 minutes or tender.

2. Mix in the scallions, garlic and cook for 30 seconds or until fragrant.

3. Add the eggs to the wok and scramble until set. Mix in the cauliflower rice and cook for 1 to 2 minutes or until the cauliflower rice is tender with a bite to the teeth.

4. Stir in the Coconut aminos, sesame seeds, and adjust the taste with salt and black pepper. Simmer for 1 minute and stir in the cheddar cheese. Turn the heat off and serve immediately.

Nutrition:

- 251 calories
- 20.68g fat
- 1g fiber

174. Wild Garlic Skillet Bread

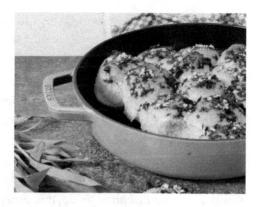

Preparation Time: 50 minutes

Cooking Time: 25 minutes

Servings: 4

Ingredients:

- 3 ¼ cups almond flour + extra for dusting
- ¼ tsp. erythritol
- ¾ tsp. salt
- ¾ oz. agar powder
- 1 cup lukewarm water
- 3/8 cup melted butter + extra for greasing
- 1 cup chopped fresh wild garlic
- Flaky salt for topping

Kitchen Equipment:

- Mixer
- Dough hook attachment
- Bowl
- Oven-proof skillet
- Oven

Directions:

1. In a mixer's bowl, using the dough hook, mix the almond flour, erythritol, salt, and agar agar powder. Add the lukewarm water and combine until dough forms.

2. Dust a surface with almond flour, add the dough and knead with your hands until smooth and elastic.

3. Brush a bowl with melted butter, sit in the dough and cover with a damp napkin. Put the bowl on top of your refrigerator and let rise for 1 hour.

4. After, take off the napkin and press the dough with your fist to release the air trapped in the dough. Divide the dough into 12 pieces and re-shape into a ball.

5. Grease an oven-proof skillet with olive oil and arrange the dough rolls in the pan. Cover with a damp napkin and let rise again for 30 minutes.

6. Take off the napkin, brush the top of the dough with olive oil, and sprinkle with the wild garlic leaves and some flaky salt.

7. Preheat the oven to 400 F/200 C.

8. Place the skillet in the oven and bake for 20 to 25 minutes or until golden brown.

9. Remove the skillet, let cool and then enjoy the bread!

Nutrition:

- 1893 calories 208.6g fat 0.7g fiber

175.Crispy Roasted Brussels Sprouts and Walnuts

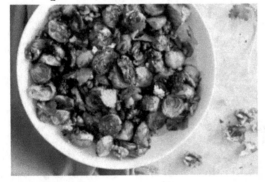

Preparation Time: 15 minutes

Cooking Time: 14 minutes

Servings: 4

Ingredients:

- 3 tbsp. almond oil
- 1/3 lb. (151.3g) Brussels sprouts, halved
- 2 garlic cloves, minced
- 1 red chili pepper, deseeded and minced
- 2 sprigs chopped fresh mint
- ¼ cup (59ml) Coconut aminos
- 1 tbsp. xylitol
- 1 tbsp. plain vinegar
- 1 tbsp. toasted sesame seeds
- ½ cup (113g) chopped toasted walnuts
- Salt to taste

Kitchen Equipment:

- Large skillet
- Bowl

Directions:

1. Heat the sesame oil in a large skillet and sauté the Brussels sprouts for 10 minutes or until softened.

2. Stir in the garlic, red chili pepper, and mint leaves for 1 minute or until fragrant.

3. In a bowl, mix the Coconut aminos, xylitol, and vinegar. Pour the mixture over the vegetables and toss well. Simmer for 1 to 2 minutes.

4. Mix in the sesame seeds, walnuts, and adjust the taste with salt as needed.

5. Dish the food onto serving plates and enjoy!

Nutrition:

- 351 calories 37.73g fat 3.93g carbs

176.Garlic cheddar Mushrooms

Preparation Time: 10 minutes

Cooking Time: 6 minutes

Servings: 4

Ingredients:

- 3 tbsp. butter
- 3 garlic cloves, minced
- 1 cup sliced cremini mushrooms
- Salt and black pepper to taste
- 1 cup grated cheddar cheese
- 1 tbsp. chopped fresh parsley to garnish

Kitchen Equipment:

- Skillet

Directions:

- Melt the butter in a skillet and sauté the mushrooms for 5 minutes or until softened.
- Stir in the garlic and cook for 30 seconds or until fragrant.
- Dish the food onto serving plates, top with the Parmesan cheese and garnish with the parsley. Serve warm.

Nutrition:

- 199 calories
- 18.27g fat
- 0.3g fiber

177.Mexican Cauli-Rice

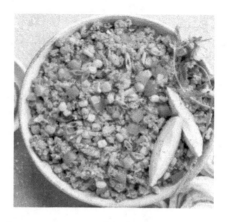

Preparation Time: 10 minutes

Cooking Time: 6 minutes

Servings: 4

Ingredients:

- 2 tbsp. butter
- 2 tbsp. almond oil
- ½ tsp. onion flakes
- 3 garlic cloves, minced
- 1 tbsp. unsweetened tomato puree
- 1 cup (227g) cauliflower rice
- Salt and black pepper to taste
- 1 cup grated Mexican cheese blend
- 2 tbsp. chopped fresh cilantro

Kitchen Equipment:

- Pot

Directions:

1. Heat the butter and almond oil in a pot and sauté the onion flakes and garlic for 30 seconds or until fragrant.

2. Mix in the tomato puree and cook for 2 minutes.

3. Stir in the cauliflower rice, add a quarter cup of water, salt, black pepper, and simmer for 3 to 4 minutes or until the cauliflower softens.

4. Stir in the Mexican cheese blend afterward and dish the food. Garnish with the cilantro and serve warm.

Nutrition:

- 223 calories
- 20.64g fat
- 0.7g fiber

178. Turnip Latkes with Creamy Avocado Sauce

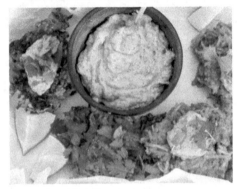

Preparation Time: 20 minutes

Cooking Time: 16 minutes

Servings: 4

Ingredients:

Turnip Latkes:

- ½ lb. (227g) turnips, peeled and shredded
- 1 tbsp. almond flour
- 1 shallot, minced
- 1 egg
- ½ cup (113g) grated cheddar cheese (white and sharp)
- Salt and black pepper to taste
- 5 tbsp. almond oil for frying

Creamy Avocado Sauce:

- ½ avocado, pitted and peeled
- 1 ½ cup (340.5g) Greek yogurt
- ½ tsp. vinegar
- 1 small garlic clove, minced
- 1 tbsp. avocado oil
- 1 tbsp. chopped fresh cilantro
- Salt and black pepper to taste

Kitchen Equipment:

- Non-stick skillet

Directions:

Turnip Latkes:

1. Place the turnips in a cheesecloth, fold up and press out as much liquid as possible. Pour the turnips into a bowl and add the almond flour, shallot, egg, cheddar cheese, salt, and black pepper. Mix well and form 1-inch patties from the mixture.

2. Heat the almond oil in a non-stick skillet over medium heat. Working in batches, add 4 to 6 patties and cook for 4 to 5 minutes or until golden brown beneath. Turn the latkes and cook the other side for 3 to 4 minutes or until golden brown too.

3. Remove the latkes onto a paper towel-lined plate to drain grease and fry the remaining patties.

Dill Yogurt Sauce:

4. Mash the avocado in a medium bowl. Mix in the Greek yogurt, vinegar, garlic, avocado oil, cilantro, salt, and black pepper.

5. Serve the latkes with the avocado sauce.

Nutrition:

- 518 calories 51.78g fat 3.6g fiber

179. Cheesy Zucchini Triangles with Garlic Mayo Dip

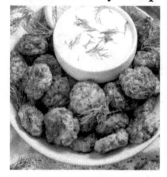

Preparation Time: 20 minutes

Cooking Time: 30 minutes

Servings: 4

Ingredients:

Garlic Mayo Dip:

- 1 cup (227g) crème fraiche
- 1/3 cup (80g) mayonnaise
- ¼ tsp. sugar-free maple syrup
- 1 garlic clove, pressed
- ½ tsp vinegar
- Salt and black pepper to taste

Cheesy Zucchini Triangles:

- 2 large zucchinis, grated
- 1 egg
- ¼ cup (20g) almond flour
- ¼ tsp. paprika powder
- ¾ tsp. dried mixed herbs
- ¼ tsp. Swerve sugar
- ½ cup (113.5g) grated mozzarella cheese

Kitchen Equipment:

- Medium bowl
- Oven
- Grease-proof paper
- Baking tray

Directions:

- Start by making the dip; in a medium bowl, mix the crème fraiche, mayonnaise, maple syrup, garlic, vinegar, salt, and black pepper. Cover the bowl with a plastic wrap and refrigerate while you make the zucchinis.

- Preheat the oven to 400 F/200 C and line a baking tray with grease-proof paper. Set aside.

- Put the zucchinis in a cheesecloth and press out as much liquid as possible. Pour the zucchinis in a bowl.

- Add the egg, almond flour, paprika, dried mixed herbs, and Swerve sugar. Mix well and spread the mixture on the baking tray into a round pizza-like piece with 1-inch thickness. Bake in the oven for 25 minutes or until golden brown and crispy.

- Reduce the oven's heat to 350 F/175 C, take out the tray and sprinkle the zucchini with the mozzarella cheese. Return the tray to the oven and bake for 5 minutes or until the cheese melts.

- Remove afterward, set aside to cool for 5 minutes and then slice the snacks into triangles. Serve immediately with the garlic mayo dip.

Nutrition:

- 401 calories 41.11g fat 0.2g fiber

180. Frozen Strawberry Yogurt Bites

Preparation Time: 10 minutes plus Freezing time: 80 minutes

Cooking Time: 0 minute

Servings: 10

Ingredients:

- ¼ cup (75g) fresh or frozen strawberries
- 2 tbsp. sugar-free maple syrup, divided
- ½ tsp. vinegar
- 2 cups (150g) Greek yogurt

Kitchen Equipment:

- Immersion blender

Directions:

1. Place the strawberries, maple syrup, and vinegar in a bowl. Use an immersion blender to process the ingredients until smooth.

2. Spoon the mixture into the holes of an ice-cube tray, halfway up. Top with the Greek yogurt to the rim of the holes. Spread out to be even and freeze for at least 4 hours.

3. Enjoy the snack ice cold.

Nutrition:

- 106 calories 10.7g fat 1g fiber

181. Bacon Cheeseburger Waffles

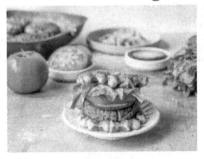

Preparation Time: 10 minutes

Cooking Time: 20 minutes

Servings: 4

Ingredients:

Toppings:

- Pepper and Salt to taste

- 1.5 oz. of cheddar cheese
- 4 tbsp. sugar-free barbecue sauce
- 4 slices of bacon
- 4 oz. of ground beef, 70% lean meat and 30% fat

Waffle dough:

- Pepper and salt to taste
- 3 tbsp. Parmesan cheese, grated
- 4 tbsp. almond flour
- ¼ tsp. onion powder
- ¼ tsp. garlic powder
- 1 cup (125g) of cauliflower crumbles
- 2 large eggs - 1.5 oz. of cheddar cheese

Kitchen Equipment:

- Skillet
- Immersion blender

Directions:

1. Shred about 3 oz of cheddar cheese, then add in cauliflower crumbles in a bowl and put in half of the cheddar cheese.

2. Put into the mixture spices, almond flour, eggs, and Parmesan cheese, then mix and put aside for some time. Thinly slice the bacon and cook in a skillet on medium to high heat.

3. After the bacon is cooked partially, put in the beef, cook until the mixture is well done. Then put the excess grease from the bacon mixture into the waffle mixture. Set aside the bacon mix.

4. Use an immersion blender to blend the waffle mix until it becomes a paste, then add into the waffle iron half of the mix and cook until it becomes crispy.

5. Repeat for the remaining waffle mixture.

6. As the waffles cook, add sugar-free barbecue sauce to the ground beef and bacon mixture in the skillet.

7. Then proceed to assemble waffles by topping them with half of the left cheddar cheese and half the beef mixture. Repeat this for the remaining waffles, broil for around 1-2 minutes until the cheese has melted then serve right away.

Nutrition:

- 18.8g protein 33.9g fats415 calories

182.Keto Breakfast Cheesecake

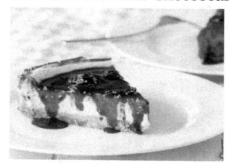

Preparation Time: 20 minutes

Cooking Time: 45 minutes

Servings: 24

Ingredients:

Toppings:

- 1/4 cup mixed berries for each cheesecake, frozen and thawed

Filling *ingredients*

- 1/2 tsp. vanilla extract
- 1/2 tsp. almond extract
- 3/4 cup sweetener
- 6 eggs
- 8 oz. of cream cheese
- 16 oz. of cottage cheese

Crust ingredients:

- 4 tbsp. salted butter
- 2 tbsp. sweetener
- 2 cups almonds, whole

Kitchen Equipment:

- Oven - Food processor
- Silicon muffin pan - Paper liners

Directions:

1. Preheat oven to around 350 F.

2. Pulse almonds in a food processor then add in butter and sweetener.

3. Pulse until all the ingredients mix well and coarse dough forms.

4. Coat twelve silicone muffin pans using foil or paper liners.

5. Divide the batter evenly between the muffin pans then press into the bottom part until it forms a crust and bakes for about 8 minutes.

6. In the meantime, mix in a food processor the cream cheese and cottage cheese then pulse until the mixture is smooth.

7. Put in the extracts and sweetener then combine until well mixed.

8. Add in eggs and pulse again until it becomes smooth; you might need to scrape down the mixture from the sides of the processor. Share equally the batter between the muffin pans, then bake for around 30-40 minutes until the middle is not wobbly when you shake the muffin pan lightly.

9. Put aside until cooled completely, then put in the refrigerator for about 2 hours and then top with frozen and thawed berries.

Nutrition:

- 12g fats 152 calories 6g proteins

183.Egg-Crust Pizza

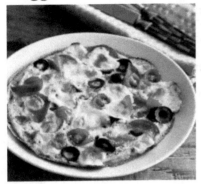

Preparation Time: 5 minutes

Cooking Time: 15 minutes

Servings: 2

Ingredients:

- ¼ tsp. dried oregano to taste
- ½ tsp. spike seasoning to taste
- 1 oz. of mozzarella, chopped into small cubes
- 6 -8 sliced thinly black olives
- 6 slices of turkey pepperoni, sliced into half
- 4-5 thinly sliced small grape tomatoes
- 2 eggs, beaten well
- 1-2 tsp. olive oil

Kitchen Equipment:

- Oven
- Broiler
- Pan

Directions:

1. Preheat the broiler in an oven than in a small bowl, beat well the eggs. Cut the pepperoni and tomatoes in slices then cut the mozzarella cheese into cubes.

2. Put some olive oil in a skillet over medium heat, then heat the pan for around one minute until it begins to get hot. Add in eggs and season with oregano and spike seasoning, then cook for around 2 minutes until the eggs begin to set at the bottom.

3. Drizzle half of the mozzarella, olives, pepperoni, and tomatoes on the eggs followed by another layer of the remaining half of the above ingredients. Ensure that there is a lot of cheese on the topmost layers. Cover the skillet using a lid and cook until the cheese begins to melt and the eggs are set, for around 3-4 minutes.

4. Place the pan under the preheated broiler and cook until the top has browned and the cheese has melted nicely for around 2-3 minutes. Serve immediately.

Nutrition:

- 363 calories
- 24.1g fats
- 20.8g carbohydrates

184.Breakfast Roll-Ups

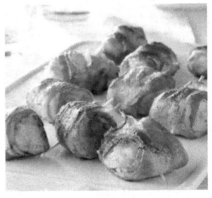

Preparation Time: 5 minutes

Cooking Time: 15 minutes

Servings: 5

Ingredients:

- Non-stick cooking spray

- 5 patties of cooked breakfast sausage

- 5 slices of cooked bacon

- 1.5 cups cheddar cheese, shredded

- Pepper and salt

- 10 large eggs

Kitchen Equipment:

- Skillet

- Whisk

Directions:

1. Preheat a skillet on medium to high heat, then using a whisk, combine two of the eggs in a mixing bowl.

2. After the pan has become hot, lower the heat to medium-low heat then put in the eggs. If you want to, you can utilize some cooking spray.

3. Season eggs with some pepper and salt.

4. Cover the eggs and leave them to cook for a couple of minutes or until the eggs are almost cooked.

5. Drizzle around 1/3 cup of cheese on top of the eggs, then place a strip of bacon and divide the sausage into two and place on top.

6. Roll the egg carefully on top of the fillings. The roll-up will almost look like a taquito. If you have a hard time folding over the egg, use a spatula to keep the egg intact until the egg has molded into a roll-up.

7. Put aside the roll-up then repeat the above steps until you have four more roll-ups; you should have 5 roll-ups in total.

Nutrition:

- 412.2g calories

- 31.6g fats

- 2.26g carbohydrates

185. Basic Opie Rolls

Preparation Time: 20 minutes

Cooking Time: 35 minutes

Servings: 12

Ingredients:

- 1/8 tsp. salt

- 1/8 tsp. cream of tartar

- 3 oz. cream cheese

- 3 large eggs

Kitchen Equipment:

- oven

- electric mixer

- cookie sheet

- parchment paper

Directions:

1. Preheat the oven to about 300 F, then separate the egg whites from egg yolks and place both eggs in different bowls. Using an electric mixer, beat well the egg whites until the mixture is very bubbly, then add in the cream of tartar and mix again until it forms a stiff peak.

2. In the bowl with the egg yolks, put in 3 oz of cubed cheese and salt. Mix well until the mixture has doubled in size and is pale yellow. Put in the egg white mixture into the egg yolk mixture then fold the mixture gently together.

3. Spray some oil on the cookie sheet coated with some parchment paper, then add dollops of the batter and bake for around 30 minutes.

4. You will know they are ready when the upper part of the rolls is firm and golden. Leave them to cool for a few

minutes on a wire rack. Enjoy with some coffee.

Nutrition:

- 45 calories

- 4g fats

- 2g proteins

186.Almond Coconut Egg Wraps

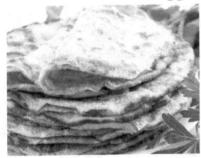

Preparation Time: 5 minutes

Cooking Time: 5 minutes

Servings: 4

Ingredients:

- 5 Organic eggs

- 1 tbsp. Coconut flour

- 25 tsp. Sea salt

- 2 tbsp. almond meal

Kitchen Equipment:

- Blender

- Skillet

Directions:

1. Combine the fixings in a blender and work them until creamy. Heat a skillet using the med-high temperature setting.

2. Pour two tbsp. batter into the skillet and cook - covered about three minutes. Turn it over to cook for another 3 minutes. Serve the wraps piping hot.

Nutrition:

- 3g carbohydrates

- 8g protein

- 111 calories

187.Bacon & Avocado Omelet

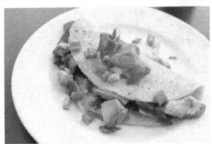

Preparation Time: 5 minutes

Cooking Time: 5 minutes

Servings: 1

Ingredients:

- 1 slice Crispy bacon

- 2 Large organic eggs

- 5 cup freshly grated Parmesan cheese

- 2 tbsp Ghee or coconut oil or butter

- Half of 1 small Avocado

Directions:

1. Prepare the bacon to your liking and set aside. Combine the eggs, Parmesan cheese, and your choice of finely chopped herbs. Warm a skillet and add the butter/ghee to melt using the medium-high heat setting. When the pan is hot, whisk and add the eggs.

2. Prepare the omelet working it towards the middle of the pan for about 30 seconds. When firm, flip, and cook it for another 30 seconds. Arrange the omelet on a plate and garnish with the crunched bacon bits. Serve with sliced avocado.

Nutrition:

- 3.3g Carbohydrates 30g protein

- 719 calories

188.Bacon & Cheese Frittata

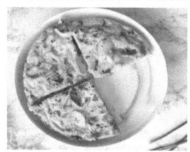

Preparation Time: 5 minutes

Cooking Time: 5 minutes

Servings: 6

Ingredients:

- 1 cup Heavy cream

- 6 Eggs - 5 Crispy slices of bacon

- 2 Chopped green onions

- 4 oz. cheddar cheese

Kitchen Equipment:

- 1 pie plate - oven

Directions:

1. Warm the oven temperature to reach 350 F.

2. Whisk the eggs and seasonings. Empty into the pie pan and top off with the remainder of the fixings. Bake 30-35 minutes. Wait for a few minutes before serving for best results.

Nutrition:

- 2g carbohydrates 13g protein 320 calories

189.Bacon & Egg Breakfast Muffins

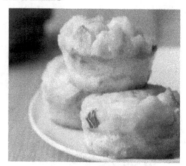

Preparation Time: 15 minutes

Cooking Time: 30 minutes

Servings: 12

Ingredients:

- 8 large Eggs - 8 slices Bacon

- 6 cup Green onion

Kitchen Equipment:

- oven

- muffin tin

- large skillet

Directions:

1. Warm the oven at 350 F. Spritz the muffin tin wells using a cooking oil spray. Chop the onions and set aside.

2. Prepare a large skillet using the medium temperature setting. Fry the bacon until it's crispy and place on a layer of paper towels to drain the grease. Chop it into small pieces after it has cooled.

3. Whisk the eggs, bacon, and green onions, mixing well until all of the fixings are incorporated. Dump the egg mixture into the muffin tin (halfway full). Bake it for about 20 to 25 minutes. Cool slightly and serve.

Nutrition:

- 0.4g Carbohydrates 5.6g protein

- 69 calories

190. Bacon Hash

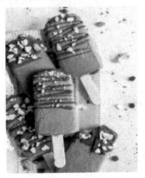

Preparation Time: 5 minutes

Cooking Time: 10 minutes

Servings: 2

Ingredients:

- 1 small green pepper

- 2 jalapenos

- 1 small onion

- 4 eggs

- 6 bacon slices

Kitchen Equipment:

- food processor

- skillet

Directions:

1. Chop the bacon into chunks using a food processor. Set aside for now. Slit the onions and peppers into thin strips. Dice the jalapenos as small as possible.

2. Heat a skillet and fry the veggies. Once browned, combine the fixings and cook until crispy. Place on a serving dish with the eggs.

Nutrition:

- 9g Carbohydrates

- 23g protein

- 366 calories

191. Fudge Ice Pops

Preparation Time: 80 minutes

Cooking Time: 0 minute

Servings: 4

Ingredients:

- ½ (13.5 oz.) can coconut cream
- 2 tsp. Swerve natural sweetener
- 2 tbsp. unsweetened cocoa powder
- 2 tbsp. sugar-free chocolate chips

Kitchen Equipment:

- Food processor

Directions:

1. In a food processor mix together the coconut cream, sweetener, and unsweetened cocoa powder. Pour into ice pop molds and drop chocolate chips into each mold. Freeze for at least 2 hours before serving.

Nutrition:

- 193 calories
- 9g carbs
- 2g protein

Ingredients:

- 1 can Stevia orange soda
- 4 tbsp. heavy (whipping) cream
- 1 tsp. vanilla extract
- 6 ice cubes

Kitchen Equipment:

- Blender

Directions:

1. Incorporate all the ingredients: in your blender and process until combines and frothy. Blend well and serve into two tall glasses.

Nutrition:

- 56 calories
- 3g carbs
- 1g protein

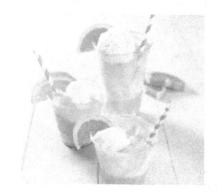

192. Orange Cream Float

Preparation Time: 90 minutes

Cooking Time: 0 minute

Servings: 2

193. Root Beer Float

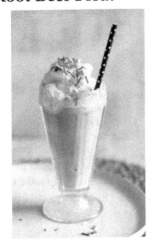

Preparation Time: 5 minutes

Cooking Time: 0 minute

Servings: 2

Ingredients:

- 1 (12 oz.) can diet root beer
- 4 tbsp. heavy (whipping) cream
- 1 tsp. vanilla extract
- 6 ice cubes

Kitchen Equipment:

- Blender

Directions:

1. Incorporate all the ingredients: in your blender and process until smooth. Pour into two tall glasses and serve.

Nutrition:

- 56 calories
- 3g carbs
- 1g protein

194. Chocolate fat Bombs

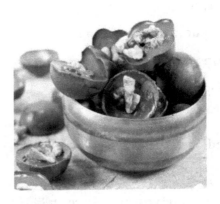

Preparation Time: 10 minutes

Cooking Time: 5 minutes

Servings: 15

Ingredients:

- 1/2 cup softened coconut butter
- 1/4 cup extra virgin coconut oil, softened
- 1/2 cup butter, softened
- 3 tbsp. unsweetened cacao powder
- 15 to 20 drops liquid stevia

Kitchen Equipment:

- Food processor
- Baking sheet
- Parchment paper
- Air fryer

Directions:

1. Put all ingredients in a food processor, storing some cacao besides for coating. Mix until smooth. Line a baking sheet with parchment paper. Make small truffles using a spoon. Situate it in the fridge for 30 minutes. Take out the baking sheet from the fridge. Put the remaining cacao powder onto the fat bombs. Set the Air Fryer at 350 F. Situate your Air Fryer basket with space in between and click air fry for 5 minutes.

Nutrition:

- 143 calories
- 2.7g carbs
- 0.9g protein

195.Coffee fat Bombs

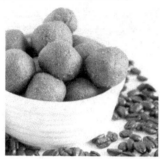

Preparation Time: 10 minutes

Cooking Time: 5 minutes

Servings: 6

Ingredients:

- 1/4 cup extra virgin coconut oil, softened
- 1/2 cup butter or more coconut oil, softened
- 3 tbsp. unsweetened coffee powder
- 15 to 20 drops liquid stevia
- *Optional*: 2 tbsp. Erythritol or Swerve, powdered
- 1 tsp. hazelnut or almond extract, or pinch of cayenne pepper
- 1/2 cup coconut butter, softened

Kitchen Equipment:

- Food processor
- Baking sheet
- Parchment paper
- Air fryer

Directions:

1. Combine all ingredients in a food processor, keeping some cacao apart for coating. Blend until smooth.

2. Place parchment paper in a baking sheet. With a spoon, make 15 small truffles. Situate it in the fridge for 45 minutes.

3. Pull out the baking sheet from the fridge. Drizzle the remaining cacao powder on top of the fat bombs.

4. Prepare Air Fryer at 350 F. Put your Air Fryer basket with space in between and select air fry for 5 minutes.

Nutrition:

- 110 calories
- 10g fats
- 21g protein

196.Berry Cheesecake fat Bombs

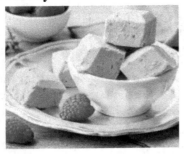

Preparation Time: 90 minutes

Cooking Time: 0 minute

Servings: 2

Ingredients:

- 4 oz. cream cheese, softened
- 4 tbsp. butter, softened
- 2 tsp. Swerve natural sweetener
- 1 tsp. vanilla extract
- ¼ cup berries, fresh or frozen

Kitchen Equipment:

- Hand mixer
- Small bowl

Directions:

1. Mix butter, cream cheese, vanilla, and sweetener using a hand mixer in a small bowl. Puree the berries thoroughly in a separate bowl. Stir in the berries to the cream cheese mixture. Transfer the mixture into fat bomb molds. Let it freeze for 2 hours and remove it from the mold. Serve.

Nutrition:

- 414 calories 9g carbs 4g protein

197.Sweet fat Bombs

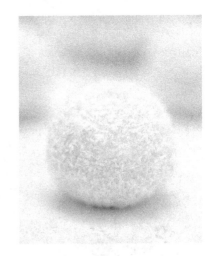

Preparation Time: 25 minutes

Cooking Time: 7 minutes

Servings: 12

Ingredients:

- 5 tbsp. Swerves
- 6 tbsp. peanut butter, melted
- ½ tsp. vanilla extract
- ¼ tsp. salt
- 6 tbsp. Erythritol
- 1 tsp. stevia extract
- 8 tbsp. fresh lemon juice
- 3 eggs
- 1 tsp. lime zest
- 2 tbsp. coconut oil

Kitchen Equipment:

- air fryer
- hand mixer

Directions:

1. Mix together the peanut butter and Swerve. Add the vanilla extract, Erythritol, and salt and beat well. Place the peanut butter mixture in truffle forms. Place the peanut mixture in the freezer. Preheat the air fryer to 350 F.

2. Mix together the stevia, lemon juice, lime zest, and coconut oil in the bowl. After this, pour the lemon mixture in the air fryer basket and cook it for 5 minutes. Stir it every 2 minutes.

3. Now, crack the eggs in the lemon mixture and mix it with a hand mixer until smooth.

4. Now, set the air fryer to 365 F and cook for 2 minutes more. Remove the curd mixture from the air fryer and refrigerate to chill. In a pastry bag, place the curd mixture. Remove truffle from the freezer. Fill each truffle with a curd mixture.

5. Place the bomb in a cold place. Enjoy!

Nutrition:

- 231 calories
- 10.3g carbs
- 3.5g protein

- Microwave

Directions:

1. In a microwave-safe medium bowl, melt the butter, coconut oil, and peanut butter in the microwave on 50 percent power. Mix in the sweetener.

2. Pour the mixture into the fat bomb molds.

3. Freeze for 30 minutes, unmold them, and eat! Keep some extras in your freezer so you can eat them anytime you are craving a sweet treat.

Nutrition:

- 196 calories
- 8g carbs
- 3g protein

198. Peanut Butter fat Bombs

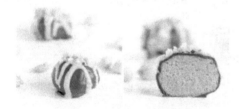

Preparation Time: 40 minutes

Cooking Time: 0 minute

Servings: 2

Ingredients:

- 1 tbsp. butter, at room temperature
- 1 tbsp. coconut oil
- 2 tbsp. all-natural peanut butter
- 2 tsp. Swerve natural sweetener

Kitchen Equipment:

199. Lemonade fat Bombs

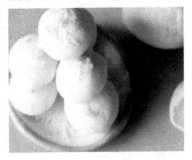

Preparation Time: 90 minutes

Cooking Time: 0 minute

Servings: 4

Ingredients:

- ½ lemon

- 4 oz. cream cheese, at room temperature
  2 oz. butter, at room temperature

- 2 tsp. Swerve natural sweetener

- Pinch pink salt

Kitchen Equipment:

- Small bowl

- Medium bowl

- Hand mixer

- Silicon cupcake molds

Directions:

1. Zest the lemon half with a very fine grater into a small bowl. Juice the half lemon into the bowl with the zest. In a medium bowl, combine the cream cheese and butter. Add the sweetener, lemon zest and juice, and pink salt.

2. Using a hand mixer, beat until fully combined. Spoon the mixture into the fat bomb molds. Freeze for at least 2 hours, unmold, and eat! Keep extras in your freezer in a zip-top bag so you and your loved ones can have them anytime you

are craving a sweet treat. They will keep in the freezer for up to 3 months.

Nutrition:

- 404 calories

- 8g carbs

- 4g protein

200. Chocolate Mousse

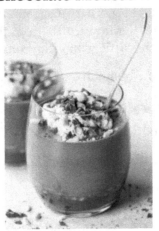

Preparation Time: 5 minutes

Cooking Time: 0 minute

Servings: 4

Ingredients:

- 1 cup creamed coconut milk

- ½ tsp. cinnamon

- Shredded coconut for garnish

- 3 tbsp. raw cocoa powder

- 6-12 drops of liquid stevia extract

Kitchen Equipment:

- Hand mixer

- Bowl

Directions:

1. Put a coconut milk can into your fridge overnight. Once thick, put it into a bowl.

Whip in raw cocoa powder. Add in cinnamon and stevia. Whip until it's smooth and creamy. Place in serving glass then garnish using some pinch of shredded coconut. Enjoy!

Nutrition:

- 218 calories
- 13.5g carbs
- 6.2g protein

Conclusion

Thank you for making it up to the end. A Keto diet provides long-term health benefits compared to other diet plans. During a keto diet, near about 75 to 90 percent of calories comes from fats, an adequate number of calories 5 to 20 percent comes from proteins, and 5 percent of calories from carb intake.

What began as a simple spark of curiosity ended on a high note: keto, which you continuously read and heard about. Now you have all the knowledge in the world to lead a lifestyle that is truly worthy of your time, energy, and effort.

A Ketogenic Diet is something that you should be starting with today for a better lifestyle if you are over 50. The ketogenic diet is more common in women than in men because of all the benefits it provides for dealing with the symptoms of menopause. Women who are experiencing menopause, or have already experienced it, have a clear idea of the troubles that come along with it. Menopause leads to fatigue, irritability, and also increases weight. But the keto diet can help in controlling your body weight and also improve your physical well-being. Are not you sure about where or how to start with keto?

Being 50 years old or more is not bad. It is how we handle ourselves in this age what matters. Most of us would have just moved on and dealt with things as they would have arrived. That is no longer the case. It is quite literally endurance of the fittest.

With keto, you are among the fittest people in existence. Your lifestyle will change dramatically, but it would be quite a pleasant change, one that you can be proud of.

Do not give up now as there will be a few days where you may think to yourself, "Why am I doing this?" and to answer that, focus on the goals you wish to achieve.

Whether you wish to stay active, lose weight, look and feel better, or any of that, keto is your solution and a way of life that will ensure you get all you need.

A good diet enriched with all the proper nutrients is our best shot of achieving an active metabolism and an efficient lifestyle. Several people think that the Keto diet is just for people interested in losing weight. You will find that it is quite the opposite. There are extreme keto diets where only 5 percent of the diet comes from carbs, 20 percent is from protein, and 75 percent is from fat. But even a modified version of this, which involves consciously choosing foods low in carbohydrate and high in healthy fats, is good enough.

The benefits are great—but those in their 40s or younger experience many of these benefits. It means that aside from the excess weight, they don't have any other health problems to contend with. But what if you're already in your 50s or more? From what I have seen, most people in their 50s already have several health issues. Usually, these are health problems that occur simply because of age—so don't feel too bad about yourself! As someone who has done extensive research and has a ton of personal experiences from working with clients, I want you to know that there is absolutely nothing to be afraid of when switching to this brand-new dietary plan.

Thanks for reading. I hope it provided you with enough insight to get you going on. Don't put off getting started. The sooner you begin this diet, the sooner you'll begin to notice an improvement in your health and well-being.

Weekly Copycat Menu

Monday	Tuesday	Wednesday
....	....	....
....	....	....
....	....	....
....	....	....
....	....	....

Thursday	Friday	Saturday
....	....	....
....	....	....
....	....	....
....	....	....
....	....	....

Sunday	Snacks	Budget
....	....	....
....	....	....
....	....	....
....	....	....
....	....	....

and up

Weekly Copycat Menu

Monday

....
....
....
....
....

Tuesday

....
....
....
....
....

Wednesday

....
....
....
....
....

Thursday

....
....
....
....
....

Friday

....
....
....
....
....

Saturday

....
....
....
....
....

Sunday

....
....
....
....
....

Snacks

....
....
....
....
....

Budget

....
....
....
....
....

Weekly Copycat Menu

Monday
....
....
....
....
....

Tuesday
....
....
....
....
....

Wednesday
....
....
....
....
....

Thursday
....
....
....
....
....

Friday
....
....
....
....
....

Saturday
....
....
....
....
....

Sunday
....
....
....
....
....

Snacks
....
....
....
....
....

Budget
....
....
....
....
....

Weekly Copycat Menu

Monday	Tuesday	Wednesday

Thursday	Friday	Saturday

Sunday	Snacks	Budget

Weekly Copycat Menu

Monday	Tuesday	Wednesday
....	....	....
....	....	....
....	....	....
....	....	....
....	....	....

Thursday	Friday	Saturday
....	....	....
....	....	....
....	....	....
....	....	....
....	....	....

Sunday	Snacks	Budget
....	....	....
....	....	....
....	....	....
....	....	....
....	....	....

Weekly Copycat Menu

Monday
....
....
....
....
....

Tuesday
....
....
....
....
....

Wednesday
....
....
....
....
....

Thursday
....
....
....
....
....

Friday
....
....
....
....
....

Saturday
....
....
....
....
....

Sunday
....
....
....
....
....

Snacks
....
....
....
....
....

Budget
....
....
....
....
....

Weekly Copycat Menu

Monday
....
....
....
....
....

Tuesday
....
....
....
....
....

Wednesday
....
....
....
....
....

Thursday
....
....
....
....
....

Friday
....
....
....
....
....

Saturday
....
....
....
....
....

Sunday
....
....
....
....
....

Snacks
....
....
....
....
....

Budget
....
....
....
....
....

Weekly Copycat Menu

Monday	Tuesday	Wednesday
....	....	....
....	....	....
....	....	....
....	....	....
....	....	....

Thursday	Friday	Saturday
....	....	....
....	....	....
....	....	....
....	....	....
....	....	....

Sunday	Snacks	Budget
....	....	....
....	....	....
....	....	....
....	....	....
....	....	....

Weekly Copycat Menu

Monday	Tuesday	Wednesday
....	....	....
....	....	....
....	....	....
....	....	....
....	....	....

Thursday	Friday	Saturday
....	....	....
....	....	....
....	....	....
....	....	....
....	....	....

Sunday	Snacks	Budget
....	....	....
....	....	....
....	....	....
....	....	....
....	....	....

Weekly Copycat Menu

Monday
....
....
....
....
....

Tuesday
....
....
....
....
....

Wednesday
....
....
....
....
....

Thursday
....
....
....
....
....

Friday
....
....
....
....
....

Saturday
....
....
....
....
....

Sunday
....
....
....
....
....

Snacks
....
....
....
....
....

Budget
....
....
....
....
....

Weekly Copycat Menu

Monday

....
....
....
....
....

Tuesday

....
....
....
....
....

Wednesday

....
....
....
....
....

Thursday

....
....
....
....
....

Friday

....
....
....
....
....

Saturday

....
....
....
....
....

Sunday

....
....
....
....
....

Snacks

....
....
....
....
....

Budget

....
....
....
....
....

Weekly Copycat Menu

Monday	Tuesday	Wednesday

Thursday	Friday	Saturday

Sunday	Snacks	Budget

Weekly Copycat Menu

Monday	Tuesday	Wednesday
....	....	....
....	....	....
....	....	....
....	....	....
....	....	....

Thursday	Friday	Saturday
....	....	....
....	....	....
....	....	....
....	....	....
....	....	....

Sunday	Snacks	Budget
....	....	....
....	....	....
....	....	....
....	....	....
....	....	....

Weekly Copycat Menu

Monday	Tuesday	Wednesday

Thursday	Friday	Saturday

Sunday	Snacks	Budget

Weekly Copycat Menu

Monday
....
....
....
....
....

Tuesday
....
....
....
....
....

Wednesday
....
....
....
....
....

Thursday
....
....
....
....
....

Friday
....
....
....
....
....

Saturday
....
....
....
....
....

Sunday
....
....
....
....
....

Snacks
....
....
....
....
....

Budget
....
....
....
....
....

Weekly Copycat Menu

Monday
....
....
....
....
....

Tuesday
....
....
....
....
....

Wednesday
....
....
....
....
....

Thursday
....
....
....
....
....

Friday
....
....
....
....
....

Saturday
....
....
....
....
....

Sunday
....
....
....
....
....

Snacks
....
....
....
....
....

Budget
....
....
....
....
....

Weekly Copycat Menu

Monday
....
....
....
....
....

Tuesday
....
....
....
....
....

Wednesday
....
....
....
....
....

Thursday
....
....
....
....
....

Friday
....
....
....
....
....

Saturday
....
....
....
....
....

Sunday
....
....
....
....
....

Snacks
....
....
....
....
....

Budget
....
....
....
....
....

Weekly Copycat Menu

Monday
....
....
....
....
....

Tuesday
....
....
....
....
....

Wednesday
....
....
....
....
....

Thursday
....
....
....
....
....

Friday
....
....
....
....
....

Saturday
....
....
....
....
....

Sunday
....
....
....
....
....

Snacks
....
....
....
....
....

Budget
....
....
....
....
....